Mental Health and Otherness

Based on two decades of research in Brazil and the UK, this book explores the ways in which intersections of gender, race and class affect the positioning of the subject as 'Other' in discourses of health and how the positioning of the subject as 'Other' has implications for health research and mental health practice.

Drawing on feminist, post-colonial and decolonial studies, psychoanalysis and discourse analysis, *Mental Health and Otherness* examines the experiences of immigrants, drug users and transsexual people in health and mental health settings and the ways in which stereotypical understandings can affect the subject.

This book is a study of the discursive construction of ideas about health and mental health in the West and the awareness of processes of othering in clinical practice. It will appeal to scholars in psychology, sociology and cultural studies with an interest in mental health, health care and intersectionality.

Ilana Mountian is Senior Lecturer in Psychology at the University of the West of England. She is a member of the School of Psychoanalysis of the Forum of the Lacanian Field and the Discourse Unit. She is the author of *Cultural Ecstasies: Drugs, Gender and the Social Imaginary* (Routledge, 2013).

Therapeutic Cultures

This interdisciplinary series explores the role which therapeutic discourses and practices play in the organisation of social life, critically addressing the two broad questions of how therapeutic knowledge is popularised beyond academia and mental health care, and how it participates in popular culture, and in institutional structures and processes in government, law, education, media, health, work, family life, public and private policies.

Therapeutic Cultures seeks to address the histories of therapeutic culture and engage with its contemporary manifestations, so welcomes books that examine the transnationalisation of therapeutic discourses and practices and their uses in local institutional settings, as well as studies of the ways in which therapeutic discourses and practices participate in the social organisation of power, and how they become ingrained across a wide array of institutions.

Titles in this series

The Dai and the Indigenous
Notes on the Appearance and Disappearance of a Figure in the Therapeutics of a Nation
Asha Achuthan

Mental Health and Otherness
Intersections between Gender, Race, Class and Age
Ilana Mountian

For more information about this series, please visit: https://www.routledge.com/sociology/series/TC

Mental Health and Otherness

Intersections between Gender, Race, Class and Age

Ilana Mountian

Routledge
Taylor & Francis Group
LONDON AND NEW YORK

First published 2025
by Routledge
4 Park Square, Milton Park, Abingdon, Oxon OX14 4RN

and by Routledge
605 Third Avenue, New York, NY 10158

Routledge is an imprint of the Taylor & Francis Group, an informa business

British Library Cataloguing-in-Publication Data
A catalogue record for this book is available from the British Library

ISBN: 978-0-367-20766-3 (hbk)
ISBN: 978-1-032-87160-8 (pbk)
ISBN: 978-0-429-26341-5 (ebk)

DOI: 10.4324/9780429263415

Typeset in Sabon
by Apex CoVantage, LLC

To my family Moissei Mountian, Sofia Mountian, Daniela Mountian, André Gal Mountian, Anatoli and Tania Mountian, my grandparents Bella and Moissei Retchester, Raissa and Iossif Mountian, Galia and Marc Katz.

Contents

Acknowledgements

Throughout these years of research and practice I have encountered a number of professionals and institutions that allowed me to research and debate fundamental issues concerning critical approaches to theory and practice in social interventions. Although I am unable to acknowledge here all my colleagues and friends who have provided important contributions and support for this work, I would like to name a few here.

Erica Burman, Ian Parker, Angel Gordo Lopes, Khatidja Chantler, Suryia Nayak, China Mills, Jemma Tosh, Barbara Biglia, David Skidmore, Ana Paula Gianesi, Elena Calvo Gonzalez, Anyky Lima, Keila Simpson, Liliane Anderson, Frederico Machado, Igor Monteiro, Marco Aurelio Máximo Prado and our colleagues from NUH/UFMG (Research group on LGBT citizenship and human rights at the Universidade Federal de Minas Gerais) and ANPEPP Gender and Sexuality Research Working Group (National Association for research in Psychology), and Miriam Debieux Rosa and fellows from the Laboratorio Psicanálise e Sociedade at the Universidade de Sao Paulo (USP).

I would like to thank Edward MacRae, Jan Simon Hutta, Ana Paula Gianesi, Angel Gordo Lopes, Erica Burman, Artemis Christinaki, Luan Cassal, Paola Ribeiro Seabra Eiras. Nadir Lara Junior and Carol Ribeirinha for their helpful comments and suggestions. Phillip Vilani for the review and suggestions. Alice Salt and Neil Jordan for kindly accompanying this writing.

Finally, I am thankful for the continuous support of my family and friends.

Introduction

On othering processes

In this book, I will seek to provide insights into key issues on the production of therapeutic cultures surrounding mental health, based on research I conducted on gender, sexuality, immigration and drug use and their impact on physical and mental health in the UK and Brazil since 1998. This manuscript ensembles previous writings on these studies. These research projects uncovered common ground and approaches for these groups. These populations were often seen as discursively positioned as the Other, with this positioning having an impact on individuals, physical and mental health care, and research initiatives. This highlights the importance of considering the social context and how intersections of gender, race, class and age operate in positioning subjects as the Other in discourse.

It is crucial to highlight that the production of otherness operates differently, although sometimes we may find similar processes, for each group (women, travestis and trans people, immigrants, drug addicts, lower classes and their intersections social categories). The impact and repercussions on these groups are fundamental to be taken into account. In this book, I will focus on the importance of critically deconstructing the ways in which specific groups are marked as the Other and question the possibilities of other subject positions.

Taking the specificities of each group into account, an analysis that encompasses the situationality of the research encounter (researcher and participants) allows for other possibilities of voice of the participant. Some of the studies undertook were able to have a thorough analysis of the position of the researcher and the participant (Mountian, 2017a), and others counted with direct participation of the interviewees in the research process (Fang et al., 2015). In this publication, some extracts of the interviews will be used in order to dialogue with the critical perspective employed. However, a deeper analysis of the relations between the researcher's positionality (cultural views, profession, gender, race and class) and the participants of the research will not be able to be further debated due to the constraints of the book length.

From these studies, I underline several issues regarding the relations between minoritised groups and mental health, focusing on two main aspects: first, how the position of the Other produced within specific social contexts

DOI: 10.4324/9780429263415-1

affects the subject's mental health, and second, a critical debate about this position of otherness and the psychological and medical perspectives on mental health, and how understanding the social context is crucial for health and social interventions. These studies highlight a therapeutic culture at play in each context, particularly focusing on the production and effects of pathologisation.

For this debate an intersectional view of minoritised groups will be undertaken, considering how social categories of gender, race and sexuality interpolate subjects, based on feminist, post/decolonial studies, discourse analysis and psychoanalysis. The main areas that will form the basis for our considerations here are immigration, women, drug use and the trans population. In these studies, we found that these groups are many times positioned as the Other in discourse, that is, through specific encounters, these groups become minoritised. The way that these groups are conceived will have a direct impact on the way that mental health is understood.

The main debates that will be explored in this manuscript relate firstly to the immigration process and its impact on mental health, and how understandings of mental health operate in relation to immigration. Secondly, we review how sexuality has been conceptualised in the medical and psychological literature, and the need for health services to consider the impact of discrimination and exclusion experienced by LGBTQIA+ people, and specificities of transgender (and LGBTQIA+) people. Thirdly, we will investigate the moral standpoints of mental health and drug use and how drug treatment and research operate according to specificities of gender, specifically for women (and intersections of class, race and age) and the impact on women and LGBTQI+ people.

Throughout these studies the othering processes of these groups were found to have a direct impact on individual health and the way practitioners treat their patients. Although these three main areas – immigrants, female drug users, and transexual people – seem distant from one another, I will focus on the production of othering processes (that occur in different ways according to each group and individual) and how particular forms of treatment are adopted (LGBTQIA+ people) or adjusted for them (immigrants, female drug users). Therefore, my focus here is on these othering processes and their effect on mental health and health care, and their impact on subjects.

Aiming to further this debate, I highlight how Othering processes can affect the treatment these groups receive in health and mental health care contexts, from not recognising the specificities of these subjects to problematic perspectives based on stereotypical understandings of minoritised groups. Particularly important for mental health are categories of normalcy and pathology. Here, either the subject's social context is ignored or a specific conception of mental health operates such that minoritised groups are constantly pathologised. This is of particular importance when considering how racial and sexual social dynamics operate over time in medicine and psy-disciplines, affecting mental health diagnoses and services. The debates presented here will consider social dynamics that are often overlooked but which risk further excluding certain social groups.

The monograph is divided into two parts: the first, 'From theory: laying foundations', outlines the theoretical background adopted to understand and deconstruct the position of the Other. The second part, 'To practice: researching mental health', presents the research undertaken and the debates surrounding the outcomes of Othering processes on mental health. The chapters that follow are adapted from previously published research and articles.

Chapter 1 sets up a theoretical debate on the (re)production and the discursive possibilities of the Other, based on discourse analysis (Foucault, 2010), psychoanalysis (Freud, 1921; Lacan, 1992), feminist (Ahmed, 2000; McClintock, 1995; Spivak, 1988) and anti-racist and post-colonial/decolonial studies (Gilroy, 2000; Balibar & Wallerstein, 2002; Fanon, 1986). This analysis highlights the discursive (re)production of the Other and how this position appears reified through fetishised relations in the debates regarding perspectives on Otherness and Sameness. The way that dynamics between the social categories operate will inform the issue of whether the subaltern can speak, and crucially, how they can be heard in psy-disciplines.

In Chapter 2, we will look at how specific socially and historically situated ideas about health and mental health in Western biomedicine and psychology have been discursively constructed. For this, we will focus on the psychiatric classifications of depression, hysteria, addiction and sexual disorders and how these classifications affect specific groups, such as women and the association with depression and hysteria; immigrants and mental health, transsexuality and homosexuality as mental health disorders; and drug addiction and minoritised groups.

The second part of the book 'To practice: researching mental health', which focuses on the above-mentioned debates based on my research conducted from 1998 until 2020, centres on three main fields: access of refugees and asylum seekers to health services in Manchester and Sao Paulo; older transwomen in Brazil; and discourses on drugs and gender in England and Brazil. These studies highlight the importance of considering the social context for the production of the Other and their effects on health and mental health practice and diagnosis.

Chapter 3 will present key aspects related to immigration and mental health in England and Brazil, focusing on issues surrounding women and young people. Analysing health policies and practices associated with immigration, fundamental issues involved in mental health diagnosis, such as the need to consider the social context of immigration and settlement, and how intersectional social categories structure the encounter between the immigrant and health service provider will be considered. I also emphasise the relevance of the immigrant's knowledge and experience in working towards decolonising practices.

Chapter 4 will further the debate surrounding mental health, focusing on issues of sexuality, based on the qualitative research with older *travestis* and transwomen in Brazil and on the study of trans people's access to education. The (in)visibility of trans people in health services and education is considered, highlighting the processes of exclusion. The older *travestis* interviewed provided historical findings regarding how transphobia impacts immigration, employment, security, education and health, particularly how trans people are considered in health and mental health services.

Chapter 5 will continue this debate, analysing how discourses related to drugs and addiction operate for female drug users. The social imaginary surrounding drug addicts will be examined, looking into how this discursive position is reproduced in treatment, drug policy and for the subject. The dynamics of intersections between gender, sexuality, race, class and age in drug policies in Brazil will be reviewed.

From these analyses on minoritising processes and mental health, questions related to ethics and diagnostics arise. In the 'conclusions' section, guided by the question 'Can the subaltern speak?' I will investigate possibilities for listening, drawing on psychoanalytic studies and unpacking the dynamics of specific power relations. This analysis seeks to create openings in discursive space for listening to the Other, focusing on such encounters so as to provide other standpoints for listening and for the discursive emergence of the subject.

Part I

From theory

Laying foundations

1 Framing the Other

This chapter outlines the main theoretical resources and debates that will accompany the reading we propose in this book. Conceptions about health and mental health are culturally and socially located forming specific therapeutic cultures. Within this, we will focus on how specific groups are 'othered', that is, positioned as different, 'unlike us'. Previous studies have highlighted how cultural and social aspects of specific groups were pathologised, for example, how mental health diagnoses were applied to immigrants (Littlewood & Lipsedge, 1989) and racialised groups (Fernando, 1988); how characteristics attributed to women, such as dependency, emotionality and infantility, are also qualities found in mental health classifications such as hysteria and depression (Allen, 1986; Mountian, 2013a); and how homosexuality was considered a mental disorder until the 1990's and transsexuality is still viewed as a mental disorder in some settings (Tosh, 2016).

It becomes fundamental to critically review how and when 'Othered' groups, such as women, LGBTTQIA+ people, black people and immigrants are assigned to mental illness (Metzl, 2010; Fernando, 1988), regarding diagnosis and the over-prescription of psychiatric medication. Two main aspects are highlighted, first, the understanding of when characteristics attributed to these groups are seen as outside of 'normalcy'; and, secondly, how discrimination, lack of recognition and social pressure affect mental health.

In order to reflect on these questions, it is crucial to examine the processes of othering of specific groups. We will do this drawing on theoretical debates around the Other from Foucault (1998), Badiou (2001), Freud (1997) and Lacan (1992); debates around the subaltern (Spivak, 1988) and abjection (Butler, 1993); and the effects of a fetishised view of the Other (McClintock, 1995; Ahmed, 2000; Burman, 2010). These debates will help us outline new possibilities for the Other in discourse, aiming to introduce other discursive avenues beyond reified views of the Other. Such possibilities instantiate the emergence of the subject, and as such, in the case studies in this book, constitute an active voice for their views on health and mental health.

DOI: 10.4324/9780429263415-3

1.1 (Re)producing the Other

Mental health research and practice face numerous challenges, from a lack of infrastructure in some countries to a lack of critical discussion that challenges hegemonic and frequently simplistic understandings of mental health. Critical perspectives in this area always find themselves in a difficult position, given that while it is important to acknowledge the effort put into offering qualified and accessible medical and psychosocial care, critical perspectives interrogate the effects of psychiatric and psychological discourses on the subject, which are necessary to further improve services and research.

From the research I have undertaken in the areas of health and mental health, particularly with drug users, trans people and immigrants, some questions emerged surrounding the encounters between minoritised groups and medical professionals. Medicalised perspectives of society are not confined to medical spaces (hospitals, universities, infirmaries) but rather structure a specific discourse that is consistently characterised as neutral and universal. Research on these encounters brings to the fore questions about how medical discourses operate in relation to Othered groups, and how they (re)produce a rather situated perspective of health and mental health.

Western medical knowledge is produced within a specific, socially and historically located epistemological tradition, and consequently carries determined views on society and subjects. The effects of this knowledge production focusing on race, class, age and gender relations, among others, can be observed in specific ways, which will be looked at in more detail in the following chapters. While we fully acknowledge the importance of medical research here, it is crucial to recognise the effects of the tacit situatedness of medical and psy-disciplines. It is essential that we critically examine tropes such as the asylum model of madness, the (moral) weakness of the drug user, the hysteria of women, the 'queerness' of LGBTQI people and the 'strangeness' of the immigrant in research and work on health and mental health. Otherwise, we risk reproducing specific discourses that continue to operate through a production of the Other. Ahmed (2000, p. 55) highlights some important aspects regarding the encounter with the Other:

> The stranger is not *any-body* that we have failed to recognize, but *some-body* that we have already recognized *as* a stranger, as 'a body out of place'. Hence, the stranger is some-body we know as not knowing, rather than some-body that we simply do not know. The stranger is produced as a category within knowledge, rather than coming into being in an absence of knowledge.
>
> (Ahmed, 2000, p. 55)

Who is the subject that medical discourse (re)produces? What knowledge production maintains the subject as a stranger, as the Other? And crucially, is it possible to listen to the Other? A number of studies have highlighted the located production of medical knowledge and the underlying risks of individualising, pathologising and psychologising the subject (Fanon, 1986; Rose, 1999; Illich, 1995; De Vos, 2013; Mills, 2014; Parker, 2011; Littlewood & Lipsedge, 1989). Therefore, feminist post-colonial and decolonial authors (Spivak, 1988; Haraway, 1988; McClintock, 1995; Ahmed, 2000; Burman, 2000; Phoenix, 1987) have highlighted the need to situate knowledge production and the (im)possibilities of listening to the Other.

First, it is crucial to question who is the Other in each specific context and how this position is structurally reproduced. Fanon (1986) defines it as the 'zone of nonbeing', arid and sterile, as the discursive location of black people in racist and colonial social structures,

> There is also the disaster of recognition. Racist imposition has made the structure one of the white self and related Other, the black self and all Others, but no white self and black Other. This below-Otherness is the disaster of black existence. It is the Zone of Nonbeing.
>
> (Gordon, 2007, p. 11)

This leaves the question of discursive space and the emergence of the subject, which will be discussed further in this chapter and in the conclusions. Here, within the production of this ontological fracture, including the intersectional production of other Others within sexist and xenophobic contexts, I return to Spivak's (1988) question regarding whether the subaltern can speak. In the following, I will focus on what psy-disciplines say about the Other, proposing an interrogation regarding how psychology and psychiatry can listen to the Other.

We can observe the medical discourses in our everyday lives from the pathologisation and psychologisation of subjects, to the formative role they play in shaping subjectivity. Rose (1994) argues that medicine is constitutively social, such that, while it needs to be understood in a social context, it also constitutes the way society has been thought about. Society, as historically produced, is accorded an organic form and thought of in medical terms. The view of society as a body produces a specific viewpoint: 'as a *social body* it is liable to sickness: that is to say, it is problematised in the vocabulary of medicine. As a social body it needs to be restored to health: that is to say, its government is conceptualised in medical terms' (1994, p. 54, original emphasis). Medicine, therefore, 'has played a formative role in the *invention of the social*' (1994, p. 55, original emphasis).

Furthermore, this view of society is far from neutral, and working from a deconstruction of medical discourses, a specific morality is observed in the definition of 'normality'. Illich (1995) analyses this moral foundation, highlighting how medicine operates as a moral enterprise, giving content to good and evil, by delimiting what is normal, proper or desirable, as law and religion do. In this way, medical discourses can operate as an ethics of life, as Rose (1994, p. 67) highlights 'our present is suffused with the ethic of the humanist, the ethic of the normal social person, which is intrinsically an ethic of the healthy body'. All aspects of care become related to the logic of health and organised around the concept of normality. In this sense, secular values of health may work discursively replacing non-corporeal or theological virtues (Katz, 1997), becoming a central ethical foundation (Mountian, 2013a).

The constitutive force of discourse has been thoroughly elaborated by a number of authors (Foucault, 1991, 2006, 2010, 1973; Parker, 1992; Burman, 2003; Fairclough, 1995; Parker & Pavón-Cuellar, 2014; Mountian, 2014a). Here, discourse is conceived as that which brings phenomenon to sight (Parker, 1992). Discourses are historically located, and it is through their specific repetition that they are instituted, that is, specific discourses gain historical fixity and solidity (Ahmed, 2000). 'Discourses are located in time, in history, for the objects they refer to are objects constituted in the past by the discourse or related discourses. A discourse refers to past references to those objects' (Parker, 1992, p. 16). Discourse analysis therefore focuses on the "different ways in which areas of knowledge and social practice are constructed" (Fairclough, 1992, p. 3). As Derrida (1991) highlights, 'writing is repeatable', that is, language can always be reiterated in a particular context and transposed into another one (Silva, 2000). This generates a focus on cultural discursive production, or as Fanon (1986, pp. 17–18) points out: 'To speak means to be in a position to use a certain syntax, to grasp the morphology of this or that language, but it means above all to assume a culture, to support the weight of a civilisation'.

Hence, there is no neutral language, which reflects the relationship between the subject and health practitioners. The importance of reflexivity for the power involved in these relations has been highlighted by feminist and anti-racist/colonial authors (Saavedra & Nogueira, 2006; Oakley, 1981; Burman, 2000; Mountian, 2017a), analysing power dynamics in these encounters and situating the subject and the medical/psychological practitioner and researcher. Here the location of the psychologist/psychotherapist/psychoanalyst is reviewed, and the relations concerning the politics of therapeutics and therapy in politics are further analysed (Frosh, 1999, 2005; Fanon, 1986; Parker, 2011; Segal, 2015; Mountian, 2015a). These crucial aspects will be further examined throughout the manuscript.

When analysing the production of the 'Other' therefore, we must situate medical knowledge and critically analyse how medicine and psychology conceive and consequently treat those positioned as the Other in discourse, and furthermore, what the dynamics of visibility and invisibility of specific social groups in health services and treatment are. Adopting Foucault's (1991) notion of the normative gaze, it is possible to interrogate how this dynamic operates with specific minoritised groups. The normative gaze refers to a form of surveillance that enables us to qualify, classify and punish. Such practices establish over individuals a 'visibility through which one differentiates them and judges them' (1991, p. 184).

We will also consider in greater detail how the Other is situated and the way groups are (in)visibilised in health services and treatment, and how this visibility repeats and mobilises specific signifiers, adopting the terms normalised absence and pathologised presence, as coined by Phoenix (1987). The way that specific groups are visibilised in mental health services and theories can be seen in the dynamics of pathologisation of the subject. Gordon (2006) highlights Fanon's conception of black psychology as discursively abnormal psychology, that is, the black person is already viewed as 'abnormal', when 'well-adjusted black' is seen as an 'abnormal', and the poorly adjusted as a 'normal black person', which means an 'abnormal person'. Such discourses reiterate the subject's 'abnormal' position, that is, the subject viewed as an Other.

In previous research on gender and drug use (Appendix 1; 2013a), we could observe how the normative gaze operates with women, where social boundaries were experienced as clearer than for men, such that transgression of these boundaries makes them more visible, producing different forms of drug taking and generating stigmatisation and ostracism. These moral boundaries were found to have specific effects on women who take drugs, such as creating obstacles to accessing health services.

It is important, therefore, to understand social categories in an intersectional manner, in specific societies and within theoretical developments. In this sense, gender is a historical construction, such that understanding gender (biologically, socially, psychically) is historically situated and constituted through intersectional processes. The intersectionality of the dynamics of social categories has, therefore, to be accounted for.

> It would be far more useful to understand how patriarchal relations articulate with other forms of social relation in a determinate historical context. Structures of class, racism, gender and sexuality cannot be treated as 'independent variables' because the oppression of each is inscribed within the other – is constituted by and is constitutive of the other.
>
> (Brah, 1996, p. 109)

The category 'woman' is seen as a shifting signifier with multiple meanings, like any other category (Henriques et al., 1984; Stacey, 1993), that is, socially and historically conceptualised, understood as performative (Butler, 1993). Therefore, the biological conceptualisation of gender requires contextualisation, wherein the biological definition of gender is historically and socially located. In this sense, the emergence of gender is an outcome of this process of construction. 'Gender is that force of reiteration of norms, the repetition of "regulatory fictions" that constitutes the subject' (Butler, 1993, p. 95), that is, it is from this reiteration that the subject is constituted. ' "Performance" is not a singular "act" or event, but a ritualized production, a ritual reiterated under and through constraint' (Butler, 1993, p. 95). Gender, in this sense, 'is the repeated stylisation of the body, a set of repeated acts within a highly rigid regulatory frame that congeals over time to produce the appearance of substance, of a natural sort of being' (Butler, 1999, p. 45). I focus here on the social expectations addressed to women in specific contexts, rather than on essentialist or prescriptive accounts. As Allen (1986, p. 104) points out,

> it is important to understand that these central problems (which are concerned, amongst other things, with issues of dependency, neediness, anger, the body, control and guilt) are not conceived simply as problems to which women are prone, but as problems to which they are prone as women.

The critical examination of how gender, race, sexuality, class and other categories operate discursively as fixed concepts, at times unrelated, and other times as undifferentiated (such as gender and sexuality), and the effects of these specific views on these categories has been thoroughly analysed and demonstrated (Rubin, 1984/2006; Scott, 1986; Laqueur, 1990; Segal, 2015).

Feminist and queer studies emphasise how bodies that do not follow the expected, linear and causal relations between sex, gender, sexual practice and desire, thereby escaping from social norms, become unintelligible (Butler, 1999). 'Gender is performed through norms of intelligibility, which are historically and culturally constructed' (Mountian, 2013a, p. 21). This expected linearity and coherence produces certain discursive effects making it crucial to interrogate the effects of discourses on gender binarism and of compulsory heterosexuality in this field (for a critique of feminist views on non-binary, gender nonconformist, trans and intersex experiences, see Tosh (2016)). Butler (1999) develops the idea of the abject when referring to sexualities outside the norm, that is, those that occupy this particular social space as unintelligible. The Other will be understood in relation to the position of the excluded and also via the constitution of the norm, that is, how the Other and we are produced through these encounters.

It is through socially and historically situated power relations that the position of the Other is (re)produced. How these power relations operate in the dynamics of visibility and invisibility of minoritised groups in each context, and in the case of this monograph, in medical and psychological services and theories, will be further examined. We will consider the experience of asylum seekers and refugees in mental health services, the view of transgenderism as a pathology and the social imaginary of women and drugs, drawing on moral ideas of purity, dependency, control, hysteria and weakness. In these examples, it is crucial to focus on how specific sexualised and racialised gazes are mobilised according to gender and its intersections with race, class, age and disability. In order to further this debate, it is relevant to focus on these dynamics related to the position of the Other within social relations that can be reiterated through fetishised relations.

1.2 Fetishised relations

A number of studies have focused on the production of the Other. Here, difference is understood as a specific value, which often oscillates between polarised discursive positions of good and bad, or more specifically between threat and victim (Badiou, 2001), or the exotic, another relevant dimension to be considered in debates surrounding otherness, wherein the Other is once again reiterated in a fixed position. Taking up the psychoanalytic perspective of the fetish (Freud, 1977a; Lacan, 1995) for the analysis of these discursive positions, a specific dynamic is revealed that involves the enchantment and fixation on the 'object' (Mountian, 2019, 2014a).

This conceptualisation has been used in diverse fields of social sciences and psy-disciplines (Mountian, 2014a). In anthropological studies, fetishism and totemism are analysed in relation to cultural and social rites (Gamman & Makinen, 1994), while for sociological studies fetishism relates to the exchange of goods. McClintock focuses on the colonial past history of fetish to analyse the intersectional relations between gender, sexuality, race and class.

In this book, I use the notion of fetish drawing on these studies aiming to provide a conceptual framework on the production of the Other in discourse, focusing on the fixed discursive position of the subject. Although the elaboration of fetishism proposed here does not follow a direct approach to each theoretical framework, it brings to the fore specific aspects that are seen as important to be accounted for a critical analysis of the social position of the Other. A subjectivist understanding of 'Marxist' fetishism is not the aim, as this would risk transforming economics into psychology. The notion of fetish proposed here is based on specific theoretical aspects focusing on the production of relations of fetishism, which, while appearing natural (to the commodity), is actually produced through human relations.

In Marx, commodity fetishism is the idea that when goods are produced for exchange, they inherit mystical qualities that go beyond mere utility ('use value'). When this happens, a disavowal of human labour occurs, displacing value to things rather than to those who produce them, thereby concealing the real social relations (of exploitation). As Marx (1990, p. 164) argues:

> The mysterious character of the commodity-form consists therefore simply in the fact that the commodity reflects the social characteristics of men's own labor as objective characteristics of the products of labor themselves, as the socio-natural properties of these things. Hence it also reflects the social relation of the producers to the sum total of labor as a social relation between objects, a relation which exists apart from and outside the producers. Through this substitution, the products of labor become commodities, sensuous things which are at the same time supra-sensible or social.

The commodity form is not solely related to the material or physical relation of the commodity, but rather to the relation among people. Fetishism comes from the 'peculiar social character of the labour which produces them' (Marx, 1990, p. 165). It is in the production process that value is created.

Zizek (1999) highlights the symbolic dimension of commodity fetishism, pointing out that in post-modernity, with the disappearance of materiality, the fetish has become even more pervasive. In his words, with 'the spectralisation of the fetish, [and] the progressive disintegration of its positive materiality, its presence becomes even more oppressive and all-pervasive, as if there is no way the subject can escape its hold' (p. 103).

In psychoanalysis, Freud developed his analysis of fetishism in relation to sexual perversions (rather than hysteria); however, he also considered that love involves a certain level of fetishism. Freud (1977a) argues that the fetish becomes pathological when it

> passes beyond the point of being merely a necessary condition attached to the sexual object and actually takes the place of the normal aim, and, further, when the fetish becomes detached from a particular individual and becomes the sole sexual object.
>
> (p. 67)

Freud outlines specific conditions for these variations and identifies a key aspect, which is the fixation on the fetish object as the possibility of *jouissance*, or its only condition of *jouissance*.

McClintock (1995) seeks to expand the conception of fetishism, understanding race and class to be as formative as sexuality. Feminist theorists have also argued for the need to revise the notion of fetishism given that traditionally it was seen as primarily masculine and phallocentric (Butler, 1993; Grosz, 1995; Rose, 1986; Apter, 1991; Gamman & Makinen, 1994). As McClintock (1995, p. 181) argues 'female fetishism dislodges the centrality of the phallus and parades the presence and legitimacy of a multiplicity of pleasures, needs and contradictions that cannot be reduced to the "desire to preserve the phallus" '.

This debate has also been explored by feminist theorists of film and culture, such as De Lauretis (1994), Mulvey (1998) and Apter and Pietz (1993). Rose (1995), for example, analysing the image of the actress as a fetish, discusses Mulvey's work on the fetishised position of the actress, highlighting how the feminine appears as a surface or facade: 'the feminised other is fetishised as a spectacle, to be looked at only as a surface concealing a lack' (p. 769). Rose (1995) argues that Mulvey shares Irigaray's critique of 'the centrality of a specific organization of a seen space to the phallocentric subject' (1995, p. 769). Similarly, it is notable how masculinity within this dynamic is positioned as powerful while the feminine is understood as passive.

The debate about female fetishism brings to the fore the discursive position of women. Irigaray claims that women cannot be the 'subject' because they are the fetish of the representation and, as such, cannot be represented, or, women cannot be represented because they are difference itself. They are not the difference or negation or the Other of the masculine subject.

> Women can never 'be', according to this ontology of substances, precisely because they are the relation of difference, the excluded, by which that domain marks itself off. Women are also a 'difference' that cannot be understood as the simple negation or 'Other' of the always-already-masculine subject. As discussed earlier, they are neither the subject nor its Other, but a difference from the economy of binary opposition, itself a ruse for a monologic elaboration of the masculine.
>
> (Butler, 1999, p. 25)

This ontological impossibility of representing women in a patriarchal society, also seen for black people in racist societies where they occupy a zone of nonbeing (Fanon, 1986), highlights the impasse of the epistemological standpoint (Spivak, 1988). While this reiteration of the ontological fissure is understood here as fundamental, I want to extend the debate regarding the fetishised production of specific social imaginaries of the subject, that I am naming here the Other. In challenging this epistemological closure, I argue for the possibility of opening up discursive fields in the analysis of the encounter. In this case, revisiting the very ambivalent character of fetishism in colonial encounters, as seen in the works of Fanon (1986), Bhabha (1994), Ahmed (2000), McClintock (1995), Hook (2012) and others.

Bhabha (1994), undertaking a reading of fetishism in Freud and of the coordination of knowledge (and power), dispositive and apparatuses in Foucault, analyses colonial stereotypes – discourses on sexuality and race – in terms of fetishism, considering the functional and structural aspects of this approach. Bhabha describes the dynamics of the stereotypical discourses of colonialism in Fanon's work *Black Skin, White Masks*, and the fetishised modes of representation in the field of identification (in Lacanian terms). The position of the Other is then reified in these fetishised relations, and it is through this discursive position that the Other becomes visible. This raises important questions regarding the effects of this dynamic on the field of mental health and health, as will be further debated throughout these chapters.

Further analysing the notion of fetish, it is significant that the term comes from the Portuguese word *feitiço* meaning sorcery, magical art, enchantment and witchcraft, derived from the Latin *facticious*, which means manufactured (Pietz, 1985). During Portuguese colonisation, *feitiço* referred to amulets and ritual objects from Africa, a term used by the Catholic priesthood in the late Middle Ages for talismans that were often illegal or heretical, coming to be related to the clerical disapproval of popular rituals.

McClintock (1995) argues that the fetish took its form during a major transformation of global economic relations, becoming a mediating object of exchange of goods and symbols. During the 18th century, 'the fetish-lands of

Africa embodied a necessary universe of errors against which the Enlightenment could measure its stately progress: errors of logic, of analytical reasoning, of aesthetic judgment, of economic progress and of political legitimacy' (McClintock, 1995, p. 187). Fetishism, following this rationale, embodied a conflict of 'cultural' values, through which Europeans could frame what was unfamiliar. As such, a negative value was attributed to what was different, so as to represent this world as deviant, inferior and negated, and creating the boundaries for what is modern. Fetishism, in this sense, provided an important discursive trope for the formation of the Enlightenment.

Following Said (1978), this view of the Other could also be interrogated in terms of Orientalism. Orientalism encompasses institutions, vocabularies and colonial styles that constitute a specific imaginary; it refers to an epistemological distinction between the Orient and the Occident. This difference is seen here as mutually reflective, 'the two geographical entities thus support and to some extent reflect each other' (Said, 1978, p. 13), though not in the same terms. In taking up this process of orientalisation, it becomes important, firstly, to critically examine the production of the Other that is put forward and, secondly, to critically analyse the notion of gender and race that is presented, as these may refer to specific situated (Western) views of gender that may differ from the way gender is locally conceived elsewhere (Oyewumi, 1997). This view of fetishism allows us to analyse the (re)production of boundaries that establish the difference. As Brah (1996, p. 117) points out '"difference as social relation" underscores the historically variable articulation of macro and micro regimes of power, within which modes of differentiation such as gender, class or racism are instituted in terms of *structured* formations'. Difference is seen according to specific values, providing specific hierarchical structural discursive positions for the construction of group identities or for the position of the Other. Difference is constituted over time, via the historical reiteration of specific discourses. Therefore, it is paramount to critically analyse how racial discourse dynamics operate, given that despite not having a biological basis, race is still prevalent in constructions of difference (hierarchical differences), 'race thinking continues' (Fernando, 2012, p. 113).

Within this production of the Other, it becomes particularly important to identify how racialised thinking interpolates health and mental health practices, and how gender and sexuality are constituted within this arena, as effects of specific dynamics of fetishisation of the Other. In colonial encounters, boundaries separating the modern and the retrograde, us and them are produced. It is possible to extrapolate geographical borders and to question the production of a domestic Other. In the research undertaken on refugees and asylum seekers' access to health services in England (Fang et al., 2015; Mountian, 2010; Fang et al., 2015) and in Brazil on immigration and mental health (Mountian, 2015b, 2020; Mountian & Rosa, 2015), discourses on immigrants reveal these discursive social positions of the Other, and more specifically of the fetishised Other.

Understanding how social constructions of gender, race, culture, class and sexuality operate is therefore crucial, considering that these boundaries are fluid and vary according to specific social and historical contexts. As such, our analysis will focus on the historical fixity of these discourses, that is, given the fluidity of these signifiers, we will interrogate the fixity of these discourses. The regime of difference that is put forward is historically reproduced (Mountian, 2019). Mills (2014) clarifies this through the work of Bhabha:

> For Bhabha (1994), one of the key facets of colonial discourse is the role of 'fixity' in the construction of otherness, with 'looking/hearing/reading as sites of subjectification in colonial discourse' (Bhabha, 1994, p. 109), where 'to exist is to be called into being in relation to an Otherness, its look' (1994, p. xvii).
>
> (Mills, 2014, p. 82)

It is therefore crucial to interrogate the colonial encounter, given its asymmetry (Ahmed, 2000), in which a production of difference encompasses a violent response. Mills (2014, p. 98) highlights how 'akin to Hook's (2005, p. 478) description of the violence of colonialism; "the colonial moment of epistemic, cultural, psychic and physical violence makes for a unique kind of historical trauma . . . [meaning that] the violence of the colonial encounter is absolutely unprecedented"'. As Ahmed (2000, p. 11) highlights: 'Colonialism as an encounter involves not only the territorial domination of one culture by another, but also forms of discursive appropriation: other cultures become appropriated into the imaginary globality of the colonising nation'. Colonisation is taken up here as this imaginary construction, not only applied to groups that 'come from afar', but also regarding how it operates within minoritised groups.

The way that discourses regarding race operate becomes central for analysing the position of the Other. Papadopoulos and Sharma (2008, p. 4) posit some key aspects about overcoming race through skin, within the situated biological production of race.

> Questioning the biological reductionism of race gives rise to post-race fantasies and the possibility of 'race overcoming' as Paul Gilroy puts it. While this position seems to be important for a vision which points beyond the tyranny of race it can neglect that racial exclusion is sustained not because it has a biological existence, but because it is literally made to have one (consider genetic screening, new databases which classify populations, genetic kinship and ancestry etc).
>
> (Papadopoulos & Sharma, 2008, p. 4)

The critical analysis of the discursive fixity on race becomes crucial, including how the concept of race is historically used (Seshadri-Crooks,

2000). As Ahmed (2000, p. 8) puts it: 'The encounters we might yet have with others hence surprise the subject, but they also *reopen the prior histories of encounter that violate and fix others in regimes of difference*'. It is within these encounters that race, and gender, are socially produced.

> Race exists insofar as capital – its conditions, relations and procedures – is spectralised, just as abstract equality exists to the extent that concrete differences are sifted, ordered, repudiated, costed and abjected. This circumstance is neither a result of will nor biology, even if it organises the semantics and practices, both mundane and sensational, of will and of bios through which race becomes materialised.
>
> (Mitropoulos, 2008)

In this sense, it is relevant to consider Balibar's notion of racism (2002, pp. 17–18):

> a true 'total social phenomenon' – inscribes itself in practices (forms of violence, contempt, intolerance, humiliation and exploitation), in discourses and representations which are so many intellectual elaborations of the phantasm of prophylaxis or segregation (the need to purify the social body, to preserve 'one's own' or 'our' identity from all forms of mixing, interbreeding or invasion) and which are articulated around stigmata of otherness (name, skin colour, religious practices).

Furthermore, Balibar (2002) questions new forms of racism, more specifically on how discourses surrounding 'culture' operate.

> It's a racism whose dominant theme is not biological heredity but the insurmountability of cultural differences, a racism which, at first sight, does not postulate the superiority of certain groups or peoples in relation to others but 'only' the harmfulness of abolishing frontiers, the incompatibility of life-styles and traditions, in short, it is what P.A. Taguieff has rightly called *a differentialist racism*.
>
> (p. 21)

Here it is important to consider how the displacement of 'race' by 'culture' operates. 'Culture' is interrogated in the way that it appears in discourse, and how the Other is reproduced in the substitution of race by culture.

This discursive dynamic has significant effects on the way immigrants are perceived. Cultural and racial discourses are closely linked and overlap, with 'culture' frequently being used as a barrier between groups, for example between asylum seekers and services providers. However, while not denying the importance of 'cultural identity' and 'cultural values', investigating how culture is spoken about, how it operates and what constitutes it is vital. In this manner, our analysis considers how culture gains meaning within encounters, taking into account specific power relations in which culture is understood as a fixed signifier. Brah (1996) defines culture as

> In broad terms, culture may be viewed as the symbolic construction of the vast array of a social group's life experiences. Culture is the embodiment, the chronicle of a group's history. Since the group histories of different sections of society differ in important ways, their 'cultures' are correspondingly different. Further, group histories are inextricably linked with the material conditions of society, so that cultures are marked by the social and economic conditions of a group at the various stages of its history. Cultures are never static: they evolve through history. That is why the process of cultural reproduction is, in part, a process of cultural transformation. . . . While the cultures of different groups in society will differ considerably, it is also the case that, in so far as at a particular point in history all groups are subjected to certain common socio-political and economic forces, they will share some aspects of one another's cultures.
>
> (Brah, 1996, p. 18)

The issue arises when difference, or more specifically cultural difference is accorded a hierarchical value. Within this, 'colonial' encounters place the Other culture in a specific imaginary position (Ahmed, 2000), often devalued, feared and/or exoticised. Considering this imaginary position occupied by specific 'cultures', it is relevant to highlight Seshadri-Crooks' (2000) analysis based on Balibar's concept of 'neo-racism', a form of racism without 'race', where 'cultural difference' has to be preserved by all possible means, thereby risking naturalising racism and overdetermining a specific genealogy, if before from 'race, now from 'culture'.

In othering processes, it is necessary to understand how minoritisation of specific others occurs through these encounters. As Chantler (2007) observes, when questioning the Other, we must question who is 'we'. While the encounter is not discursively symmetrical, being produced within specific power relations, nonetheless, it produces both the difference and possibilities of transformation. As Ahmed (2000, p. 11) argues 'colonial encounters involve a necessarily unequal and asymmetrical dialogue between once distant cultures that transform each other'.

Race and culture appear as having specific functions in discourse, in this case, that of reiterating specific positions of the Other. It becomes paramount to interrogate and challenge these differences based on a social imaginary of race and culture. Within this debate on the racialised Other, how intersections between gender and sexuality are (re)produced and performed in contemporary contexts, and particularly in medical and psychological practice, must be recognised, as these relations can be obscured, ignored or pathologised.

1.3 Celebrating difference: on otherness and sameness

It is crucial for us to understand how the discursive position of the Other is produced for clinical practice and public policy. This position reveals discursive polarisations between I and Other, Us and Them, a difference that carries social value. In the research with immigrants and health (Appendix 1; Mountian, 2015b, 2020), we can observe how the immigrant is often viewed as a victim, a threat and/or exotic, limiting the discursive possibilities of the subject positioned as a fetishised Other. Spivak (1988) questions, 'Can the Subaltern Speak?' Considering the hegemonic epistemological limitations (and violence) of the standpoint location, what are the possibilities of listening the Other?

> The clearest available example of such epistemic violence is the remotely orchestrated, far-flung, and heterogeneous project to constitute the colonial subject as Other. This project is also the asymmetrical obliteration of the trace of that Other in its precarious Subjectivity.
>
> (Spivak, 1988, p. 76)

In this debate, Spivak (2010, p. 83) defends the need for representation of the subject without mediation: 'If, in the context of colonial production, the subaltern has no history and cannot speak, the subaltern as female is even more deeply in shadow'. A number of aspects related to representation become important here: the acknowledgement of minoritising processes, the importance of a politics of representation and the effects of difference taken as an essentialist dimension. This brings to the fore the debate on identity politics as a political strategy rather than an ontology of the subject (Butler, 1999). As Crenshaw (1994, p. 94) points out:

> The problem with identity politics is not that it fails to transcend difference, as some critics charge, but rather the opposite – that it frequently conflates or ignores intra group differences. In the context of violence against women, this elision of difference is problematic, fundamentally because the violence that many women experience is often shaped by other dimensions of their identities, such as race and class. Moreover, ignoring differences *within*[1] groups frequently contributes to tension *among* groups, another problem of identity politics that frustrates efforts to politicize violence against women. Feminist efforts to politicize experiences of women and antiracist efforts to politicize experiences of people of colour have frequently proceeded as though the issues and experiences they each detail occur on mutually exclusive terrains.

Another aspect regarding representation refers to the epistemological divisions between society and the individual. Parker highlights some aspects of this in the debate between Butler, Laclau and Žižek in *Contingency,*

Hegemony, Universality: Contemporary Dialogues on the Left (2000) on the antagonisms between the social and the individual, positioning the antagonism at the level of representation.

> The deadlock of representation that each of them worries away at opens the way, perhaps, to break from a notion of the individual and social as separate and instead to attend to this deadlock as a constitutive aspect of the social and as constitutive of the individual subject. Antagonism 'between' the individual and the social is then one manifestation of the deadlock of representation rather than its original defining source. Žižek makes the point most explicitly in his argument, against Laclau, that the antagonism is 'internal' to the subject and the social rather than operating 'between' the two.
>
> (Parker, 2003, p. 1)

This deadlock in speaking of the subject (and 'our' listening) is our focus in this work. Focusing here on immigration and refugee policy, while these can be extended to other public policy areas, I further investigate two key discursive strategies: celebration of difference (otherness, multi-culturalism) and the politics of sameness, 'we are all the same'. These strategies will serve here to illustrate a debate towards listening to the Other. While we recognise here the importance of these strategies in specific moments and contexts, I analyse them broadly, seeking to outline the discursive binaries produced. These approaches seem to oscillate between polarised views that can reinforce the fetishised position of the Other.

Debates on multi-cultural and anti-racist policies brought up important aspects for consideration. Anthias and Yuval-Davis (1996) analyse some of the educational policies from 1980s in the UK and USA, highlighting elements for anti-racist approaches, pointing out on the one hand, the risks of ongoing power imbalances, and on the other hand, the hazards of maintaining the essentialisation of specific groups. Among a number of questions, they analyse how the notion of community and race operate in these settings. Taking up the notion of community in multi-culturalist and anti-racist approaches, they point out that discursively 'the multiculturalist notion of the community based on culture, and that of anti-racism on colour' (Anthias & Yuval-Davis, 1996, p. 162). Keeping these debates in mind, I look at these discursive divisions between sameness and otherness in discourses on the immigrant.

Regarding the celebration of the Otherness in discourses on 'cultural difference', Zizek (1998, p. 168) critiques how they can constitute an ambiguous relationship with racism. As I stated earlier, I do not deny cultural differences nor the importance of certain initiatives that attempt to situate these differences in other discursive positions; however, it is important to maintain a critical analysis in relation to such interventions to avoid reiterating the subject within fetishised relationships. Such a critical analysis can look at how 'difference' appears in discourse, as on the one hand a celebration can ignore the very differences, while on the other, it can maintain the place of the Other, rather than interrogating the production of these differences when socially diminished in discourse.

Zizek (1998, p. 168) comments:

> Without the real of jouissance, the Other remains ultimately a fiction, a purely symbolic subject of strategic reasoning exemplified in the 'rational choice theory'. For that reason, one is even tempted to replace the term 'multiculturalism' with 'multiracism': Multiculturalism suspends the traumatic kernel of the Other, reducing it to an aseptic folklorist entity.

Zizek (1998, p. 168) continues quoting Michaels (1992, pp. 682–685): 'Our sense of culture is characteristically meant to displace race, but . . . culture has turned out to be a way of continuing rather than repudiating racial thought'.

It is important, therefore, to note that the notion of race is embedded within multi-culturalist discourses. Hence, race and culture appear to have specific functions in discourse; in this case, they can work to reiterate specific positions of the Other, rather than questioning the production of these differences based on race/culture.

Regarding the strategy of sameness, 'we are all the same', while I also start from the understanding that we should all have the same rights, we must recognise that groups do not occupy the same social position or access the same rights. Overlooking this may risk ignoring the unequal power positions that these groups occupy in discourse, thereby erasing social differences. Badiou (2001) critiques perspectives based on a self-evident character of the human condition, highlighting two key aspects. Firstly, on the production of polarised views on the debate, and secondly, about how the victim position can operate here. How people are victimised should obviously be acknowledged; however, there is an aspect in these discourses that demands further analysis, particularly when a specific performance of the victim is expected within these discourses for the subject to access their rights, and finally, guaranteeing rights only when the other is viewed as a 'good' other. Within the debate surrounding the notion of 'difference' and a 'right to difference', Badiou (2001) argues that the ethics of human rights seem to define an identity such that respect for the different is given to those who are 'reasonably consistent with this identity' (p. 24). Badiou (2001, p. 24) asks: 'the celebrated "other" is acceptable only if he is a good other (- which is to say what, exactly if not the same as us?)'. This adds another dimension that involves identity and representation.

Taking up the critique from Butler (1999, p. 9) on the identity of 'women' as defined by *the* feminist movement: 'the identity of the feminist subject ought not to be the foundation of feminist politics, if the formation of the subject takes place within a field of power regularly buried through the assertion of that foundation'. In fact, the debate on identity is as already stated crucial, not as a fixed notion, but rather, through questioning how and when it functions as a fixed signifier, and on the political strategy for social solidarity (Gilroy, 2000). In this direction, we can critically interrogate how immigrants, for example, can at times be expected to have to fulfil an identity prescribed, based on specific discourse also seen in human rights campaigns (human rights campaigns are very important!), as a specific performance, that is that of the victim, not allowing for other discursive positions. A number of authors have critically analysed this specific imaginary. Fassin and Rechtman (2009), for example, extend this debate through an analysis of discourses on trauma and victimology looking at the individualising and psychiatric use that can depoliticise or decontextualise the subject's suffering. Burman (1999) critically analyses the images of children in charity and humanitarian campaigns and the discourses mobilised in these images.

In the 'we are all one' discursive strategy, there is a possibility, therefore, that the Other is only considered one of us, when s/he is a 'good other, that is, the same as us'. There may also be a danger of erasing social-historical differences, as highlighted by Ahmed (2000, p. 16) 'an ethics that responds to each other as if they were other in the same way is inadequate'.

This is an important discussion for both public policy and everyday discourse, noting an oscillation between the celebration of otherness and a celebration of sameness. In any case, it is important to ask when/if the immigrant (or the asylum seeker) continues to occupy this reified position, while the possibility of (self) representation and possibilities of ambiguity and desire of the subject are obliterated. I will highlight some of these aspects in public policy throughout this manuscript and in the final remarks. Moreover, this debate also involves the notion of community that underlies these perspectives. As Anthias and Yuval-Davis (1996, p. 190) point out 'a new definition and interpretation of the areas of culture and community is, from this point of view, necessary, in order to transform them into sites of positive resistance'. This is of particular importance for immigrants and 'other Others', when seen as bodies out of place (Ahmed, 2000).

When discourses are fixed via these dichotomic perspectives in public policy and public discourse (sameness and otherness), there are not many other discursive possibilities for the immigrant, who is, in any case, either positioned as the Other as in multi-culturalism (also exoticised in the celebrations), or in terms of sameness, where either structural positions are ignored, or s/he is incorporated as a 'good other', that is, the same as us.

So, in this sense, it is crucial to identify the symbolic position of the asylum seeker and the immigrant in discourse, which frequently oscillate in public discourses between the positions of victim, threat or exotic. This social imaginary is analysed according to social-political contexts, the socio-historical production and reproduction of discourses, that can continuously reify the immigrant in the fetishised position of the Other, or provide other discursive spaces. As Ahmed (2000) points out: 'To talk of the migrant as the stranger is not sufficient. It cannot deal with the complexities of the histories, not only for the displacement of peoples, but the demarcation of places and spaces of belonging' (Ahmed, 2000, p. 79). In this sense, it is crucial to look at the historical determinations of estrangement, without assuming an ontology of the stranger.

Furthermore, there is a critique of post-colonial and/or decolonial approaches, which claim that debates about the in between and hybridity can be complicit with dominant power relations (see Ahmed, 2000; Painter, 2015). However, the focus here is on how these discourses operate in relation to the production of the Other, in the analysis of how the image of the Other or the stranger figures within globalisation and multiculturalism debates, the construction of boundaries, and the place that hybridity and in-betweeness occupies within these (Ahmed, 2000).

In this debate, it is fundamental to consider how the social categories of gender, sexuality, race, age, disability and class operate within specific social contexts. This raises important analytical challenges: What are the dynamics of these categories? What is the discursive position occupied by immigrant women? How is sexuality dealt with and recognised in public policy? And finally, is there a discursive space for the Other to be seen as a subject? Ahmed (2000, p. 6) suggests that to avoid the 'fetishism of the stranger'

> by examining the social relationships that are concealed by this very fetishism. That is, we need to consider how the stranger is an effect of processes of inclusion and exclusion, or incorporation and expulsion, that constitute the boundaries of bodies and communities, including communities of living (dwelling and travel), as well as epistemic communities.

It is crucial to interrogate the power relations that underlie these encounters in order to widen the space for other discursive positions of the Other, towards an emergence of the subject.

1.4 Working with intersections

Building up on the production of the position of the Other it becomes crucial to analyse the encounter. Ahmed (2000, p. 6) points out: 'I describe such processes in terms of encounters in order to show how there are determined, but not fully determined. The term encounter suggests a meeting, but a meeting which involves surprise and conflict'. It is through encounters that the 'us' and 'them' divide is produced, and it is also through encounters that change can be thought. This presents a number of challenges for critical analysis and for the deconstruction of a perspective characterised by discursively fixed positions. The work on intersectional categories that interpolate the Other becomes paramount for critical research.[2] In this sub-section, I focus on the debates surrounding intersectionality and reflexivity.

Intersectionality

An awareness of how ideas about 'Otherness', entrenched within specific power relations, intersect with gender, race, class, age, disability and sexuality at a local, on-the-ground level, is central to a comprehensive understanding of how groups are perceived in public policies and health care provision.

Intersectionality has already been established as a key notion for critical theory and social intervention (Burman, 2005; Crenshaw, 1994; McClintock, 1995; Berger & Guidroz, 2009). There are, however, numerous ways to approach intersectionality, particularly in its on-the-ground implementation, producing tensions and debates within and between academic forums and social interventions. Intersectionality has long been an important aspect within critical feminisms (Beauvoir, 1949/1993; Lorde, 1980/1997; Sedgwick, 1991; Benhabib & Cornel, 1987; Yuval-Davis, 1997; hooks, 1984/2005), challenging the traditional academic and lay understanding of social categories as universal and neutral (Haraway, 1991; Butler, 1999). Rather, this approach to intersectionality emphasises that social categories are situated and relational (Haraway, 1991; Chantler, 2007; Burman, 2005; Brah & Phoenix, 2004; Crenshaw, 1994).

While some feminist scholars defend the importance of accounting for 'women' as a category in academic analyses, others, both from within the academy and social movements questioned the production of essentialist notions of woman (Keller & Longino, 1996; Harding, 1986; Butler, 1999). Here, the debate focused on the importance of incorporating the discussion on gender in academic spaces, while critically questioning how the notion of woman was used. This provides a challenge for research and practice, that is, the importance of deconstructing mainstream understandings of what it is to be a 'woman', whilst maintaining the inclusion and recognition of the specificity of gender according to the social context and local struggles, both within academic circles, as well as in public policy and social work.

The recognition during the second wave of feminism of how the category 'woman' was a socially constructed category, and that 'women' were not inferior to men, had a crucial impact in a number of academic settings in several countries (Berger & Guidroz, 2009; Saavedra & Nogueira, 2006). This dynamic was also present in social movements, particularly during the 1970s both in Europe and the US, and in countries from the Global South, such as Brazil, with struggles towards women's autonomy, labour rights and increased presence in politics. Nonetheless, a specific and restrictive understanding of the category woman was still in play. This limitation was raised by Black Feminists (Lorde, 1980/1997; hooks, 1984/2005; Mohanty, 1994; Nayak, 2015); Marxist Feminists (Benhabib & Cornel, 1987; Federici, 1975; Haraway, 1988); Post-Colonial, decolonial and Subaltern Studies (Segato, 2006; Gonzalez, 1984; Shwarcz, 1993; Spivak, 1988; McClintock, 1995; Vergès, 2020); Feminist Queer studies (hooks, 1984/2005; Butler, 1999; Lorde, 1980/1997); and Crip Studies (McRuer, 2011), as well as by diverse social movements (the so-called third wave). The differences and the invisibility of diverse groups of women were highlighted, producing important critiques of the universal understanding of the category 'woman', influencing how history, politics and science were understood.

In the case of Brazil, this process of contesting women's social position was linked to wider processes of political change, struggling for general political rights, as well as more specific demands from parts of organised civil society such as anti-racist initiatives from organised Black Women's movements, LGBTQI+ movements and grassroots organisations[3] (Saffioti, 1969/2013; Alves & Pitanguy, 1991; Gonzalez, 2020; Rago, 2013; Facchini, 2009; Prado et al., 2010; Damasco et al., 2012; Carneiro, 2003; Facchini et al., 2020). Debates around representation and identity politics have been seen in both academic and activist settings in Brazil (Hollanda, 2019; Gonzalez, 2020; Saldanha & Nardi, 2016; Machado et al., 2017).

These debates are important for the Brazilian context, where there is still a need for feminist, anti-sexist and anti-racist perspectives in public policy, despite the development of public policy initiatives over the past 20 years. Amongst these, we can highlight the creation of projects to criminalise violence against women, programmes that aim to combat homophobia, LGBTQIphobia and sexism in schools, and the implementation of racial quotas in a number of universities. It is relevant to point out that these initiatives are not completely established and face opposition from certain political sectors and religious fundamentalist groups, particularly evangelic ones, as seen, for example, in the resistance to implementing anti-sexist and anti-LGBTQIphobia projects in schools (Correa et al., 2021; Mountian, 2013b). In fact, by the time this manuscript was written, several governmental backlashes can be seen directly affecting public policy to protect minoritised groups (Correa et al., 2021).

Feminist and anti-racist studies and activism have highlighted the ways in which power relations operate according to gender, race and other social categories that are taken as fixed in discourse (Haraway, 1991; Butler, 1999; Fanon, 1952/2008; Balibar & Wallerstein, 2002; Appiah, 1992; Mbembe, 2001). Contemporary debates on women concede that, while there is no universal category of woman, in patriarchal societies gender-based oppression still operates at diverse levels (Butler, 1999). Therefore, the intersectionality proposed by Black feminism, queer, and anticolonial feminist debates is one that defies an essentialist view of woman, however, accounting for the imbalance in power relations in specific social contexts (Burman, 2015; Butler, 1999).

While there are various ways to approach intersectionality, a critical view of these inter-related categories is understood here as necessary. We highlight how some of these debates have been put forward in post-colonial settings, and imply another level of analysis, highlighting the importance of considering the dynamics of colonial heritage. In particular, the specificities of how power relations operate within post-colonial contexts accounting for the colonial past and its contemporary discursive repetition.

Understanding colonial history within the Brazilian context has proven to be a challenge for academic research and social movements. Studies have emphasised the importance of taking into account Brazilian history when analysing how intersections between race, gender and class operate in this context, revealing how discourses reproduce and maintain specific social positions (Carneiro, 2003; Gonzalez, 1984; Nascimento, 2003; Shwarcz, 2012; Santos et al., 2012; Munanga, 1990; Santos, 2000; Schucman, 2014; Ribeiro, 2016; Damasceno, 2018); nonetheless, there is still a need for critical research on the intersectionality of colonial relations and their current discursive reproduction within the matrix of domination (Hill Collins, 2000, p. 18).

Research and analysis that focuses on intersecting social categories is a constant challenge, given that while it is fundamental to consider unequal social categories for the analysis, it is crucial to remain critically vigilant to avoid hierarchisation, reification, essentialisation and relativisation of social categories. Therefore, we highlight two debates here: one on identity politics and the other on the structural production of social categories.

Anthias and Yuval-Davis (1996, p. 192) argue that Rosalind Brunt's observations regarding 'the issue of representation' are the starting point for any politics of identity. They emphasise two aspects in their debate: How identities are represented and assigned to specific categories, and who represents the groups politically? This brings to the fore how politics operate within these categories, a question that has been central in feminist debates.

The expression 'the personal is political' coined in the 1970s, broaden the notion of politics, no longer restricted to governmental politics, but also embracing the politics of everyday life. Here, I would like to highlight two points in relation to 'the personal is political'. Firstly, how everyday life and the body also become political, and secondly, regarding the political representation of women and LGBTQI+ people. Mouffe (1998) differentiates between the political and politics. The political refers to social relations, and politics to the sphere of governmental politics.

> By 'the political', I mean the potential antagonism inherent in social relations, antagonism which can manifest itself in many different forms. 'Politics' refers to the ensemble of discourses, institutions and practices whose objective is to establish an order, to organise human coexistence in a context that is always conflictual because of the presence of 'the political'. Politics is concerned with the formation of an 'us' as opposed to a 'them'. It aims at the creation of unity in a context which is always one of conflict and diversity
>
> (Mouffe, 1998, p. 16)

Silvia Federic (2013)[4] highlights how, starting from the history of feminist movements and struggles, there has been a redefinition of the political and a refusal to equate it solely with the sphere of government and the law, thereby expanding the political to the everyday, the personal, family and domestic relations, and to daily relations. The personal is political encapsulates this re-definition. Citing the slogan of women in Chile in the 1970s and 1980s: 'Democracy in the home, democracy in the country', meaning one cannot separate the democratisation of relations in the family, that is, the reproductive relations, from the democratisation of political power in general. Federici (2013) argues that the feminist movement has unveiled critical aspects of capitalism, showing how the separation between public and private was instrumental in hiding the unpaid work done by women. Federici points out the devaluation of reproductive labour, and the resulting control over women's finances and bodies. The political character of the home is brought to the fore.

The political nature of the body, of those aspects that are commonly seen as private or domestic, is crucial for feminist and queer studies. How power relations operate within/between bodies is described and challenged. Rubin (1984/2006, p. 144) argues that

> The realm of sexuality also has its own internal politics, inequities, and modes of oppression. As with other aspects of human behaviour, the concrete institutional forms of sexuality at any given time and place are products of human activity. They are imbued with conflicts of interest and political manoeuvres, both deliberate and incidental. In that sense, sex is always political. But there are also historical periods in which sexuality is more sharply contested and more overtly politicized. In such periods, the domain of erotic life is, in effect, renegotiated.

It is crucial to acknowledge how the body is sexually marked (Beauvoir, 1949) and the effects of this. The politics of the body, the dynamics of identity politics and the effects of coming out have been amply discussed by numerous authors (Sedgwick, 1991; Warner, 1999; Butler, 1999). In *Epistemology of the Closet*, Sedgwick debates dynamics of identity politics (from a non-reductionist perspective) and sexuality (e.g., LGBT, Jewish), critically reading the social dynamics of sexual binary systems and the power asymmetry in Western cultures, focusing on the politics of the closet (the politics, effects and ways of coming out).

> As Foucault says: 'there is no binary division to be made between what one says and what one does not say; we must try to determine the different ways of not saying such things. . . . There is not one but many silences, and they are an integral part of the strategies that underlie and permeate discourses.' 'Closetedness' itself is a performance initiated as such by the speech act of a silence – not a particular silence, but a silence that accrues particularity by fits and starts, in relation to the discourse that surrounds and differentially constitutes it. The speech acts that coming out, in turn, can comprise are as strangely specific. And they may have nothing to do with the acquisition of new information.
>
> (Sedgwick, 1991, p. 3)

Therefore, the recognition and inclusion of a politics of the body, the everyday, and their effects on the subject is fundamental, while also understanding the ontology of the subject conceived as open, that is, not taken as a fixed and limiting category. The importance of identity politics and the risks of taking it as a fixed category have been debated by numerous scholars (Butler, 1999; Crenshaw, 1994; Mountian, 2017b).

These intersectional categories operate within specific social contexts, which constitute the way these categories are viewed and valued in discourse. As such, how patriarchal societies conceive gender and sexuality has a direct impact on the way groups are positioned socially. For feminist psychoanalysts, patriarchy works at all levels (conscious and unconscious). As Stacey (1993, p. 57) notes, 'feminist work on the psychic dimensions of patriarchy has explored ways in which the broader structures of society operate within kinship relations in the formation of individual identities'. The debate between psychoanalysis and feminism, which I cannot engage with here, is extensive (Mountian, 2015a; Gianesi & Mountian, 2019); nonetheless, the aspect we will consider, which is central for our inquiry, is how women and LGBTQIA+ people are often discursively positioned as the Other.

This discursive positioning of the subject effects the way that medicine and psychology understand specific groups, which can reproduce unequal differences. Further, it is worth highlighting how a view on institutional racism affects the way that groups are conceived. As Fernando (2012, p. 116) observes:

> 'Institutional racism' [was] a concept first proposed in the 1960s by Stokely Carmichael and Charles Hamilton (1967) in Black Power, to explain educational and social disadvantage in the US. But it is only since the Macpherson report (Home Department, 1999) blamed institutional racism for failures of the Metropolitan Police (the police department in London, UK) that it has come into mainstream discourse in the UK vis-a-vis psychiatry and the mental health services. Macpherson defined institutional racism as follows:
>
> > The collective failure of an organisation to provide an appropriate and professional service to people because of their colour, culture or ethnic origin. It can be seen or detected in processes, attitudes and behaviour which amount to discrimination through unwitting prejudice, ignorance, thoughtlessness and racist stereotyping which disadvantages minority ethnic people.
> >
> > (1999, p. 28)

These socially constructed dynamics are reproduced and operate in everyday life, raising the question about how we can critically approach these intersecting categories given that we too are also located within these social dynamics. Feminist studies emphasise the importance of situating knowledge (Haraway, 1988) and call for ongoing critical reflexivity (Burman, 1998).

Reflexivity

Reflexivity is a tool that was used by some feminist researchers in order to highlight and reflect upon the embodied and institutionalised power relations of the researcher. It is part of the process of critical research, raising questions about the researcher's position in the field, and regarding how this impacts both the analysis and the subject's approach to research questions (Mountian, 2017a). Nogueira (2001, p. 50) defines research reflexivity as: 'the critical and public evaluation of the process and the interpretative resources'.

Considering the reflexivity of the researcher and practitioner requires a critical analysis of the positions taken for granted within the research context and how power relations operate within these dynamics. This is an ongoing process, as different discursive layers appear in relation. Foucault's (1998) views on power allow us to identify some of these power dynamics, as power is not related solely to domination or to forms in which power is instantiated. As such, it is not simply a structure or institution, 'it is the name that one attributes to a complex strategical situation in a particular society' (Foucault, 1998, p. 93). Power is related to the process, 'the multiplicity of force relations immanent in the sphere in which they operate, and which constitute their own organization' (1998, p. 92). As a process, through struggle, changes and the support these forces give to one another, they constitute a system. Or, they can appear in isolation, arising as the strategies through which they take place (e.g. the state apparatus, law). This would be 'power's condition of possibility, or in any case the viewpoint which permits one to understand its exercise' (1998).

As discussed elsewhere (Mountian, 2017a), the inclusion of an approach to power relations in research is difficult, given that on one hand it requires a constant *reflexivity* from the researcher, and on the other, it may expose the researcher who responds to a 'scientific' community that demands 'objectivity' as the grounds for 'well-executed' research. Further, reflexivity involves acknowledging the researcher's standpoint from a number of angles, including the institutional setting, the researcher's social position according to intersectional social categories such as gender, race, class, age and sexuality, and the epistemological and methodological perspectives they adopt (Haraway, 1988; Harding, 1986), including their ethical implications (Parker, 2005). These elements are incorporated into the research allowing for a critical analysis, considering the relation between the subject and the researcher and practitioner.

Perhaps here we can utilise the psychoanalytic terminology of transference (Freud, 1912, 1913), where the focus is on the analyst-analysand relationship, while still comprehending the power relations implicit within transference. I will present further reflections on this point regarding resistance and listening in the final chapters.

Many feminists call for the inclusion of reflexivity (Harding, 1996; Stanley & Wise, 1990), as well as an 'interpretive vigilance' (Burman, 1998) in research and practice. Based on her research on pregnant women, Oakley (1981) debates the difficulties and contradictions in research and the limits of the research process, which requires a further reflection about how questions are structured. Some of the aspects Oakley highlights are the importance of a non-hierarchical position, engaging with interviewees, and the effect of interviews on the subjects (in this case, participants talked about the therapeutic effect that the interview produced). The impact of the interviews on the participants should be carefully considered; as in some circumstances, the questions might trigger difficult memories, and in others, the researcher's position of authority might generate specific effects for the participants and for the research (for example, as seen in the research with immigrants).

This makes clear the impossibility of neutrality on the part of the researcher and practitioner, and the risks of (re)producing power relations, even unintentionally, given that knowledge is always situated. Our goal here will be to recognise the position of the subject and the research, such that the focus becomes the encounter between the researcher and the participant, and the possibilities of maintaining and/or transforming both discursive positions.

1.5 Encountering the Other

> 'Borders are set up to define the places that are safe and unsafe, to distinguish *us* from *them*.'
>
> (Anzaldúa, 1987, p. 3)

Centring on the encounter, it is important to ask how the Other is constructed and crucially to identify who is the Other in these constructions. Taking on Ahmed's analysis on anti-racism, some insights emerge. 'Anti-racism requires interventions in the political economy of race, and how racism distributes resources and capacities unequally amongst others' (Ahmed, 2004, p. 12). It is in the encounter that it becomes possible to perceive this distribution. However, a question remains: What are the discursive possibilities of the Other? This is relevant when the subject is placed in the discursive position of Other and is consistently seen as part of a homogeneous group identity where idiosyncrasies, paradoxes and dilemmas are overlooked.

In earlier studies (Mountian, 2017a, p. 159), it was seen that, 'We can be multiple, different, with different wishes and desires, while They can only be what We imagine of Them. Reflecting on this reification of the Other in discourse, the non-conformal positions can be seen as providing a space for the emergence of the subject. The importance in recognising the social position in which the subject is placed, without reducing the subject into one only imagined identity, into an ontology of the Other'.

The Other is then viewed as a fetishised Other, which again leads us to the question 'Can the Subaltern Speak' (Spivak, 1988/1994). Spivak argues on the subaltern's impossibilities of to speak in relation to hegemonic listening, highlighting the deadlocks and debates stemming from epistemic, imperial, disciplinarian and social violence. The subaltern is defined by difference.

Spivak underlines how the subaltern is obliterated in sexual difference, since the construction of gender reproduces patriarchal forms of domination, 'the woman is doubly in the shadow' (Spivak, 1988/1994, p. 84).

This fetishisation of the Other is commonly seen at every level of social interaction. How this appears in mental health, however, is the main question considered here, focusing on the production of the Other in psy-disciplines, requiring a constant reflexivity for the critical work.

The need to take intersections between gender, sexuality, race, class, age, religion (Littlewood & Lipsedge, 1989) and disability (Grech, 2011, 2015) into account for critical work and analysis raises a number of questions and challenges. Some particularly pressing aspects include considering these intersectional categories; acknowledging the researcher's and practitioner's standpoint; situating these within the social context; and crucially, accounting for the encounter between the researcher and the subject, and more broadly, between 'us' and 'them'. The encounter with the Other can be seen as a site for the reproduction of established power relations, as well as for transgression and transformation. 'It is fundamental then to consider how power operates in the processes of regimes of difference, the borders instituted and the roots of passage, which posit the subject as the Other, in the encounter with Us' (Mountian, 2017b, p. 160). Taking up Brah's (1996) conception of border in both a geographical and analytical sense, we can ask how borders are produced within encounters.

> Borders: arbitrary dividing lines that are simultaneously social, cultural and psychic; territories to be patrolled against those whom they construct as outsiders, aliens, the Others; forms of demarcation where the very act of prohibition inscribes transgression; zones where fear of the Other is the fear of the self; places where claims to ownership – claims to 'mine', 'yours' and 'theirs' – are staked out, contested, defended, and fought over.
>
> (Brah, 1996, pp. 194–195)

It is through encounters that difference is produced, and the value accorded to the Others is constituted, which directly affects the subjects and the encounters themselves. It is in the encounter that identity is produced; although not fixed, these are often assumed as such, as the repetition of specific signifiers produces a mark in how the subject is viewed. Therefore, the discursive possibilities of the Other become restricted, when caught up in pre-given, stereotypical conceptions to which they are subject. Listening to the Other requires a continuous reflexivity, an interrogation through the encounter and of the encounter. Still, how can we listen to the Other, of more precisely, to the fetishised Other?

Adding another dimension to this debate, in Spivak's account of the subaltern's possibility to speak, and analysing the dynamics of race-gender-class-Third World categories in discourses about Hindu women, Spivak asks, what is the woman's desire? Spivak presents an analysis about how power, desire and politics are intricate and heterogeneous, emphasising the importance for critical analysis of recognising the subject's desire.

The social imaginary of the Other when reified and homogenised commonly negates the desiring subject, that is, the dynamics of power and desire are not recognised for the Other. As Spivak (1988/1994, p. 68) argues 'when the connection between desire and the subject is taken as irrelevant or merely reversed, the subject-effect that surreptitiously emerges is much like the generalized ideological subject of the theorists'. What was the Hindu widows' desire regarding the law and the tradition of self-immolation upon her husband's death? What were the power relations at stake? This also brings to the fore the idea that the recognition of the Other's desire can provide space for the Other to be seen as a subject. In terms of the research presented here, what are the desires and voices of the women, LGBTQIA+ people and immigrants regarding service provision and the public policies focused on them?

> But what does it mean to speak for those who have been refused access to reason and knowledge, for us who have been regarded as mentally ill? With what voice can we speak? Can the jaguar or the cyborg lend us their voices? To speak is to invent the language of crossing, to project one's voice into an interstellar expedition: to translate our difference into the language of the norm; while we continue, in secret, to practise a strange lingo that the law does not understand.
>
> (Preciado, 2020a, p. 20)

Maintaining these interrogations is important for critical research that seeks to reflect on the possibility of representing the subject without mediation (Spivak, 1988). Our analysis, therefore, focuses on the dynamics of power and desire from the subject's perspective, and the possibilities of challenging a reified and homogenised view of the Other. What is the subject's desire? What are the discursive possibilities for the emergence of the subject? If it is through the encounter that the Us and Them is mutually constituted, we assume that the encounter can also produce change. Other perspectives that adopt counter-hegemonic or non-hegemonic discourses highlight how tensions and dilemmas that challenge binary traps can make available other discursive positions for the subject (Halberstam, 2011). Moreover, the psychoanalytic notions of desire and transference can provide insights for this debate, which I will further develop in relation to some aspects of the encounter, seeking to apply these psychoanalytic resources in the concluding remarks of this manuscript.

Key aspects

This chapter aimed to set up the theoretical approach to the understanding of the production and positioning of minoritised groups as the Other in discourse, focusing on the dynamics of the fetishisation of the Other. We set up the key resources to deconstruct and challenge gender, sexuality, race and class divides, as well as the view of structural power relations regarding these categories. From this, we argue on the possibilities of producing alternative discursive spaces for the emergence of the subject, in that the desire of the Other is considered. Within this, it is a claim that while the encounter produced the division Us and Them, it is also through the encounters that it is envisaged possibilities of change and discursive opening.

Notes

1 Italics in the original
2 This sub-section is based on Mountian, I. and Gonzalez, E.C. (2019). 'Reflections on the theory and practice of intersectionality: immigration and health provision services in Brazil', p.92–104. In Nayak, S. and Robbins, R. (eds). Intersectionality in Social Work: activism and practice in context. London: Routledge
3 For further insight into these issues, see https://www.youtube.com/watch?v=KbWQQsO5kAY
4 http://www.youtube.com/watch?v=enpTFJsswWM

2 Mental health classifications and othering processes

On addiction, depression and sexual disorders

This chapter outlines critical theoretical debates on mental health and otherness, focusing on three main psychiatric classifications: the notion of drug addiction, depression and transsexuality. For this, we will explore critical debates on the development of mental health classifications and the effects of social constraints on people's health. Our focus on these classifications emphasises how an understanding of the Other is operative in the area of mental health. While the debate centres on these particular classifications, it also invites us for a continuous critical analysis in psychological and psychiatric practice and research.

This analysis uncovers the effects of discourses on mental health and therapeutic culture in terms of three main aspects: how specific groups were pathologised; how mental health disorders operate in relation to marginalised groups; and how certain groups were historically seen as embodying specific mental health diseases. While assuming the vital role of mental health support for individuals, we claim that a careful analysis of these discourses can firstly guarantee adequate care according to the specificities of each subject, and secondly, provide a context to interrogate how particular discourses operate to reproduce the marginalisation and stigmatisation of specific subjects and groups. This marginalisation occurs due to individualised and pathologised perspectives, neglecting the effects of the social context and interpolation by intersectional categories of gender, race, class, age, sexuality and disability.

Firstly, we will explore mental health and gender considering how medical discourses on women's physiology, particularly on hormones and emotions, pathologised women. For this, I will engage with debates surrounding depression and the consequent over-prescription of anti-depressants for women, highlighting how medical discourses reveal and reproduce certain specific conceptions of women (Ettorre, 1992). This debate can encompass other groups as well, such as immigrants, considering the interplay of intersectional social categories of gender, race and age.

Secondly, extending this debate, diverse forms of sexual identity and practices have been historically viewed as mental disorders, codified in mental health classifications of homosexuality and transexuality (Missé &

DOI: 10.4324/9780429263415-4

Coll-Planas, 2011). This foregrounds the importance of the contemporary discussion surrounding the impact of this diagnosis on LGBTTTQIA+ people.

Thirdly, we will present a historical overview of how drug addiction came to appear in psychiatric classifications in Western societies, becoming an emblem for any behaviour seen as compulsive (Sedgwick, 1992; Katz, 1997), emphasising the limits and contradictions of this conception, and how it affects specific groups, such as women, the working class, immigrants and black people, in terms of particular forms of drug use.

The relations and effects of medical discourse on minoritised groups have been well documented by critical authors (Foucault, 2006; Rose, 1999; Mills, 2014; Fernando, 1988; Littlewood & Lipsedge, 1989). Adopting a feminist, post-colonial and decolonial perspective, the analysis of the intersectional categories of gender, race, class, age, disability and others presents challenges as it makes available views on the (re)production of power relations in medical and psychological discourse regarding their effects on the treatment and care of minoritised subjects, providing critical tools for health practice and theoretical debates.

To interrogate some of these key discursive operations, it is crucial to bear in mind the importance of the medical discourse in the production of social discourses and the constitution of subjectivity. Numerous authors have underlined the impossibility of a neutral and universal medical discourse (Haraway, 1991; Harding, 1986; Foucault, 1973); rather, these frameworks must be historically and socially situated for the analysis of the effects of discourses on the production of subjectivity and knowledge (Parker, 1992; Hacking, 2006).

It is in the 19th century that we can locate the turning point for the rise of medical institutions, which came about in dialogue with religious discourses and governmental organisations (including law enforcement). Hence, the knowledge produced by medicine cannot be seen in isolation from its context, and in this sense, it becomes important to identify and analyse the (re)production of specific moralities.

As Rose (1994) observes, the 19th century established various apparatuses associated with health. These did not concern only medical practice, but rather were related to the public sphere more generally for fighting diseases. Additionally, the domestic sphere was subject to scrutiny and regulation on the basis of medical terms. During the 20th century, these medical and health regulations entered schools and work places, transforming them into 'inspection machines' (1994, p. 63), establishing institutions for old, young and disabled individuals. This regime provided a new rationality in which security needed to be maximised through risk management.

> Medicine, the paradigmatic profession that has most successfully defended its privileges, knowledge base, and monopolistic control, established itself at the top of the professional hierarchy in the early years of the twentieth century and has remained there since. Nineteenth-century medicine was weak, divided by secretary claims, rife with

> cranks; its status was middling, somewhere beneath that of the law; its practitioners were a motley lot, encompassing on the one hand a genteel, college-educated, European-trained elite and on the other men (and some women) in far greater numbers whose skills were informally acquired through the unregulated means of apprenticeship and short medical courses.
>
> (Lunbeck, 1994, p. 27)

Medical and pharmaceutical institutions, as we understand them today, were established and regulated throughout the 20th century. This was a period during which psychiatric knowledge and practice were thoroughly constituted. For the analysis of the development of medicine and the expansion and of this knowledge production (advancements), knowledge of the body and remedies (epistemology), and its separations and stigmas (politics), Foucault's work bring important critical historical perspectives. The traditional methodology of history searches for continuity, repetitions of series and the effects these produce. Foucault (2010) argues for a deconstruction of such an approach, where what is at stake is not a 'total' history, but rather, a 'general' history, by which the aim is to

> determine what form of relation may be legitimately described between these different series, what vertical system they are capable of forming, what interplay of correlation and dominance exists between them, what may be the effect of shifts, different temporalities, and various rehandlings, in what distinct totalities certain elements may figure simultaneously.
>
> (Foucault, 2010, p. 11)

This makes explicit the importance of an analysis that apprehends the discontinuities, disruptions and what remains unsaid, when identifying dominant or hegemonic discourses. In this sense, a critical reading considers the social power relations and the effects of these discourses. For example, the history of medicine, while appearing neutral, when closely examined reveals the emergence of a specific ethics that produces particular understandings. Hence, what is called medicine is produced within a 'series of associations between events distributed along a number of different dimensions, with different histories, different conditions of possibility, different surfaces of emergence' (Rose, 1994, p. 50).

Foucault (2010) highlights how medicine in the 19th century was characterised by a style, a specific way of formulating statements. Here, medicine inaugurated 'a corpus of knowledge that presupposed the same way of looking at things' (2010, p. 36), which divides, analyses and describes phenomena. Medical discourse came to refer to a specific ethics of life, regulations, models and descriptions. The clinical discourse carries an epistemological value, and it provides intelligibility (Osborne, 1994).

From 1800 psychiatry began to define differences in definitions for mental illness. The alienist identified the mentally ill, isolated them and subsequently reintroduced them to society. In the 1830s, the medical profession and psychiatry became more clearly defined. At the time, psychiatry was a practice separated from medicine. The psychiatrists, known as 'alienists', worked in asylums, coming to occupy a key position for the diagnosis and classification of pathologies that defined if the person was ill, insane or in need of care. Punitive practices were analysed by several authors, highlighting the moral and religious frameworks informing medicine during this period (Lunbeck, 1994). Psychiatry came to replace religious perspectives regarding what is normal and abnormal.

Littlewood and Lipsedge (1989) highlight how before the 19th century, people displaced from rural areas during early capitalism, formed an itinerant population of dispossessed peasants, who were often condemned as heretics or witches. In France, diverse groups such as criminals, the unemployed and the mentally ill, who were confined together, all came to be categorised as mentally ill.

The moral foundations of medicine and psychiatry explored by Foucault (1974/2012) were embedded in the production of a specific 'truth' seen in the treatment of the sick and insane. Many of these perspectives are still in play in a variety of practices and diagnoses, from the young to the elderly, establishing what is normal. Maintaining a disciplinary approach from an asylum perspective, they also operate as social control, a political device (Moncrieff, 2010). Furthermore, diagnoses produce a mark on the subject and their family, such that anomaly and madness become discourses that can stigmatise whole families. 'If anomaly leads to madness and if madness produces anomaly, it is because we are already inside this collective support that is the family' (Foucault, 1974/2012).[1]

Definitions of anomaly are located socially within the encounter between medicine and the Other. Furthermore, within this production, it is crucial to question the tacit presuppositions through which specific groups are already situated as outside the norm, and as such, in need of control, including women, LGBTQI+ people and immigrants. As Laqueur highlights:

> More generally, biology and human sexual experience mirrored the metaphysical reality on which, it was thought, the social order rested. The new biology, with its search for fundamental differences between the sexes, of which the tortured questioning of the very existence of women's sexual pleasure was a part, emerged at precisely the time when the foundations of the social order were shaken once and for all.
>
> (Laqueur, 1990, p. 22)

The moral underpinnings of medicine and its use for social control since the 19th century have produced specific effects on minoritised groups. Fernando

(2012) points out how this view of mental illness is operative in relation to colonisation and globalisation:

> Containment of 'criminality' and/or 'mental illness' – the social control of people judged as requiring custody because they were mentally ill although often apprehended for activities that were deemed 'criminal' – went hand in hand with medical approaches towards helping people deemed to suffer from mental illness.
>
> The situation in non-western cultural traditions of (say) Asia, Africa, and pre-Columbian America is very different. But during colonialism, and even more so as a part of more recent 'globalisation', western beliefs about mental health and illness and ways of controlling the latter have been imposed and/or taken up across most of the world (see Watters, 2010).
>
> (Fernando, 2012, p. 114)

Two aspects are significant here: firstly, how mental health classifications can affect specific groups, and secondly, how the social situatedness of understandings of health and care; in this context, the encounter with the Other shows that conceptions of health are heterogeneous, disclosing the ethical presuppositions of medicine. Fernando (2012) highlights a difference stemming from the individualistic view of the subject, arguing that in many non-Western mental health contexts there is an emphasis on the harmony and stability of the outer world of relationships in contrast to the individualistic perspectives of individual autonomy and self-esteem found in the West.

Moreover, in modern psychiatry, there is an attempt to diagnose mental illness in the same way as physical illness, which in fact are not equivalent (Moncrieff, 2010). A critical deconstruction of the ethical and moral grounds of medicine, psychiatry and psychology allows us to perceive the effects of classifications and the importance of considering the situated specificities and differences for the medical and psychological practice.

2.1 Women and mental health: on depression and hysteria

It is fundamental to consider how medical and psychiatric frameworks are socially and culturally situated, most specifically within the Western context. Although this seems well known, particularly when we consider past experiences in medical practice and diagnostics, it is still the case that the effects of these discourses on everyday practice are frequently present and not fully acknowledged in current theories and practices. The formulation of mental health diagnoses cannot be separated from a socially and historically situated understanding of 'normality' (Foucault, 2006). As such, it becomes necessary to analyse how mental health classifications were developed alongside the pathologisation of specific minoritised groups. In this section, we look at the production of mental health disorders, especially depression and hysteria, focusing on discourses about women, through the intersectional lens of categories of gender and race.

In this analysis, I will firstly explore how discourses on madness operate in relation to women, and how specific aspects of madness interact with discourses about what is expected from women, that is, how characteristics expected from 'normal' women (e.g. docility, infantility, emotionality) are those attributed to madness, producing specific effects on women and a feminisation of mental illness. Secondly, I will extend the debate regarding how the diagnosis of depression and hysteria affects minoritised groups in diverse ways, from over-diagnosis to the individualisation of issues that are in fact socially grounded. In previous studies on drug use, gender and race (Mountian, 2005, 2013a), we can see how discourses on addiction and other mental health issues commonly posit the subject as a victim of biological and/or psychological functions, thereby separating the individual from the social context. As claimed earlier, we do not ignore mental health suffering; however, acknowledging how classifications operate is important to avoid increasing suffering and risking alienating the subject from their own history and social relations.

The feminisation of mental illness reveals how discursive characteristics of women are posited as 'abnormal', and why people who are psychiatrically diagnosed are often treated as infantile, intellectually limited and emotionally unreliable, converging with the way that women are seen and treated in specific contexts.

Critical analyses of the discursive position of women as the Other (sex) (Beauvoir, 1949/1993) have been thoroughly developed by a number of feminist studies (Butler, 1999; Burman, 2000; Spivak, 1988). Warner (1996) highlights how the signifier 'madness' discursively functions by marginalising women, as ill, 'somehow second rate', the second-sex. Furthermore, these discourses produce a concept of madness 'as fearful, as individual, as invariably feminine, as sickness' (Ussher, 1991, pp. 11–12).

'Natural madness' and the 'vulnerability' of women were traditionally ascribed to female biology (Allen, 1986), with Western medicine portraying women as closer to nature (including their reproductive functions), to contradiction, unpredictability, amorality and madness. Madness for women was associated with the realms of nature and sexuality (e.g. via menstruation), with the brain said to be driven by instincts (both sexual and maternal). This contrasts with men, in whom madness was regarded as a consequence of deviance from socially attributed masculine roles (Engel, 1997). These ideas are reflected in women's traditional social roles associated with the domestic sphere (children, marriage and natural motherhood). In this manner, female physiology was transformed into 'a cultural rationale which assigns women to nature and the domestic sphere, and thus ensures their general inferiority to men' (La Fontaine *apud* Littlewood, 1994, p. 78).

The way that gender figures in the field of biology and medicine, particularly in how women's bodies were thought in terms of hormones and a consequent inability to work, have been challenged (Preciado, 2020a; Rohden, 2003; Saavedra & Nogueira, 2006). Common-sense ideas about women's bodies and psyches as fragile, and guided by maternal and sexual instincts, also contributed to lesser social position for women. For example, in 1910, Thorndike (quoted by Hollingworth, 1914, p. 510) stated: 'if men differ from each other in intelligence and energy through greater extremes than women, the highest and leading positions in the world must inevitably belong to men. They will deserve them more often'[2] (Saavedra & Nogueira, 2006, p. 15). This idea places women in a lower position in terms of work, while it considers the male body as the reference for medicine.

Up until the 18th century, medicine was based on the male model, that is, the epistemic concerning gender difference was situated. As Laqueur (1990) claims, when differences were established, they were already embedded in gender power relations, such that interpretation of the body becomes the result of epistemological and political developments.

While emotionality is expected from women, this signifier can also operate by characterising women as incapable of coping with social responsibilities, reproducing an old emotion-reason opposition. This view of emotions can have effects on the analysis of women, such as the association with hysteria, while insufficiently emotional women may be viewed with suspicion, possibly as (sexually) 'deviant'. This social imaginary of emotionality has a specific impact on the idea of madness, as the latter is often related to the uncontrollability of emotions. Littlewood (1994, p. 84) in the analysis of advertisements for tranquilisers underscores how women are portrayed as suffering from 'diffuse emotional symptoms' while men experience 'discrete episodes of anxiety'. These 'male' symptoms are seen as provoked by specific circumstances of pressure at work or by a physical disease, different to women, whose symptoms are related to their 'nature'.

Hockey (1993, p. 254) argues that 'the apparently ungendered profile of madness – passivity, emotionality, irrationality, dependency, lack of initiative, and need for support – is also a profile of a "normal" woman'. This brings to the fore a discursive field for gender within mental health, in which the socialisation of women meets categories of mental illness, with women who do not correspond to this expectation being placed in a 'marginal' position. As such, more independent women or those who present more aggressive behaviour compared with social expectations may risk other psychiatric diagnoses, such as psychopathy or personality disorder.

'Badness' or aggression were seen as 'incompatible elements of the female psyche, femininity implied a fragile vulnerability that required a vigorously aggressive husband/protector' (Haaken, 2002, p. 8). Furthermore, it is crucial to investigate how this image applies to working class women, black or immigrant women who were frequently characterised as deviating from 'femininity'. The direct impact on how sexuality operates will be further analysed in terms of discourses about drug addiction in Chapter 5.

In this sense, madness can also function by replacing badness (also found in other discourses on drugs), different to men, whose aggressiveness is more socially acceptable. Warner (1996) highlights the haste in applying the label of madness to women who break the law, as women are more likely to be detained in psychiatric divisions than men are in the criminal system.

It is relevant to consider in greater detail how specific psychiatric classifications were associated with and applied in relation to women. Here I will focus on debates surrounding hysteria, sado-masochism and depression, and in Chapter 5, on drug addiction. In the 19th century, hysteria was considered a female characteristic, a 'perverse femininity' (Littlewood, 1994). At the end of the 19th century and the beginning of the 20th, women were confined in hospital facilities in very high numbers, sometimes permanently, with treatments including a series of painful methods.

During the 17th and 18th centuries, 8000 indigent women were placed in Salpêtrière hospital in Paris, the largest hospice in Europe, later including prostitutes, disabled people and epileptics (Mathon et al., 2018). The women ranged from 15 to 30 years old. 'The typical patient was the eldest of a large number of children (5–12). In spite of herself and very early on, she became a substitute mother and had to witness little brothers and sisters dying from convulsions and fevers' (Walusinski, 2014, p. 66). Many lived in poverty and were sexually harassed or abused by their employers. Patients presented physical symptoms (convulsions, speech problems, sudden mood changes) and sexual 'anomalies'. The conditions of the hospitals and the treatment prescribed for the patients were appalling.

> Imagine rows of several dozen beds, some closed off with curtains to hide the 'reposantes', prostrate patients who were often incurable. Heating during the winter was inadequate, provided by only a few stoves. Visitors were suffocated by pestilential odours.
>
> (Walusinski, 2014, p. 65)

The association of women and hysteria provoked intense reactions. The 'mystery' attributed to women produced particular effects in this context, with the 'mysterious' woman evoking both romantic and paranoid fantasies, seen in ideas such as aggression coming from her seductive tactics: 'violence lies in her charms' (Gay, *apud* Haaken, 2002, p. 9). Moreover, women who defied gender expectations and women activists in the feminist movement could also be diagnosed as hysteric (Showalter, *apud* Tosh, 2016). The way medical diagnosis replaced religious discourse regarding women and 'deviance' can be seen from previous instances such as 'witchcraft' to 'mental illness' (hysteria) (Tosh, 2016).

Hysteria, from the Greek *hysteron* meaning womb, relates to early ancient Greek ideas of the 'disorder' caused by a 'wandering womb', a consequence of not bearing children, and in the Middle Ages, due to 'excessive' sexuality.

Treatments included surgeries in the ovaries and uterus (Tosh, 2016). From the 16th century onwards, theories started to look at the nervous system or mind for an explanation (Tosh, 2016). The way that treatment was conceived for women has been criticised, following punitive and reclusive treatment.

> Briquet's (1859) *Traite de l'Hysterie* (Treatise on Hysteria) was based on the study of 430 individuals, and highlighted sexual 'excessiveness' and low social class as causal factors for 'hysteria' (also known as 'Briquet's syndrome'), in addition to youth and being a woman. Consequently, he recommended changes in social conditions for treatment (Mai & Merskey, 1980, p. 1401). This was in stark contrast to Weir Mitchell's (Mitchell, 1875, 1904, 1908) influential bed-rest cure, which included seclusion, no activities, a loss of autonomy over basic tasks such as eating, and has since been compared to solitary confinement (Ussher, 1992). Mitchell described his treatment of 'hysteria' as follows: 'She was put to bed, and left it for no purpose. At first she was fed and washed by others, and forbidden to read or use her hands, and even to talk' (Mitchell, 1875, p. 95).
>
> (Tosh, 2016, p. 30)

By the 19th century, ideas about hysteria started to change. Charcot's work in the late 19th century started to include the diagnosis of men, although women were the ones mostly diagnosed. Breuer and Freud, through their work with Anna O., presented another perspective in relation to treatment, proposing listening to the subject and taking the speech of women (and men) into account, focusing on free association and repressed memories. This approach to women can be regarded as a turning point for treatment, moving from 'physiology' to 'psychology'. Regarding the psychoanalytic method, it is important to highlight that it requires a constant reflexivity, as it is also not exempt from silencing or ignoring women's voices. A number of debates have taken place regarding the possibilities of psychoanalytic listening (Van Haute & Geysken, 2016; Tosh, 2016; Parker, 2011). I will return to this question in the final chapter.

Despite the critiques and changes in psychiatric diagnosis, it is worth asking how hysteria still figures in everyday discourses and psy-discourses (Mountian, 2015a). This discursive construction can be seen, for example, in the haste in diagnosing women as hysterics, or the everyday utilisation of the word 'hysterical' for women. Moreover, studies have highlighted how some contemporary diagnoses carry characteristics similar to hysteria, such as 'histrionic personality disorder' that is still utilised; borderline personality disorder, mostly applied to women and considered the 'new' female malady, this disorder is considered vague and contradictory (Tosh, 2016); and anorexia nervosa that has been seen as a successor diagnosis for hysteria in women (Ussher, 2018).

Feminist theorists have produced a number of studies on the effects of diagnosis on the subject, and call for an analysis of the production of symptoms that considers the social context. In this sense, the social position of women has to be considered for the analysis of how hysteria and other forms of distress (e.g. depression) can be interpreted, which, in specific societies, can also signal the undervalued social position of women. In this sense, the symptom can also be seen as a form of resistance, of coping and/or reaction. Moreover, moving from an individualised and isolated understanding of the symptom to a social one can provide further insight. Gould (*apud* Tosh, 2016) emphasises how dislocating the reading of 'histrionic personality disorder' from an individual conception of mental illness to an awareness of the implicit social dynamics can provide a comprehension of the symptom as a 'cultural disorder', that is, as 'a result of attitudes toward traditionally feminine styles of interaction' (Tosh, 2016, p. 26), as one way for women to respond to a 'disordered culture'. The symptom, therefore, also manifests the need to understand structural social dynamics.

Studies have demonstrated specific correspondences between individual diagnosis and social conditions, such as the relations between the label 'hysteria' and the socially devalued place of women; findings regarding the diagnosis of 'borderline personality disorder' where many women with this diagnosis had been sexually abused (Ussher, 2018); and 'self-defeating personality disorder' which potentially framed victims of domestic violence as 'mentally ill' (Tosh, 2015, p. 12). Ussher (2018) has also argued that how hormonal and sexual disorders appear in psychiatric diagnosis is another important area of research, wherein female behaviour is pathologised and judged, such as 'female sexual dysfunction' and 'premenstrual dysphoric disorder'.

Another contested diagnosis is that of masochism, which when applied to women ignites another important debate, as women are often seen as 'naturally' masochist, representing a pathological form of feminine love. Masochism was named after the author Sacher-Masoch from his book *Venus in Furs* in 1870, and sadism from the novels of Sade. To Masoch's displeasure, Kraft-Ebbing named a 'perversion' after him (Beckmann, 2009), initially defined as the 'association of passively endured cruelty and violence with lust' (Tosh, 2016), opposed to sadism, where pleasure would be the result of inflicting pain and humiliation. These categories are considered to some degree as 'normal', and when going beyond a certain point, as pathological, for the DSM, as a 'sexual deviation' and subsequently as 'paraphilia.

The discourse on the natural passive role attributed to women can be seen in the formulation of this mental illness, 'as Krafft-Ebing (1895) explained, "Owing to her passive *rôle* in procreation and long existent social conditions, ideas of subjection are, in women, normally connected with the idea of sexual relations"' (Krafft-Ebing *apud* Tosh, 2016, p. 36). The association between sexuality and passivity was viewed as 'an instinctive inclination to voluntary subordination to man', which was 'often accepted with secret satisfaction' (2016, p. 138). This positioning of women as naturally passive and (secretly) desiring domination by male partners permeates the work of Ellis, who highlighted their 'complementary structure' (2016, 36).

This association between women and masochism raises several important issues for further analysis, including in relation to discourses around domestic violence. The position of masochism as passive also has to be further interrogated. While sadism is typically understood as active, and therefore representing a male stereotype, masochism is viewed as a feminine, passive characteristic, a "sign of impotence" (Beckmann, 2009, p. 40). Moreover, several debates concerning the social construction of S&M and power relations have been undertaken (Beckmann, 2009; Demaj, 2014). Beckmann (2009) contests the classification of S&M as a mental illness, as it stigmatises the subject and semi-criminalises consensual practices, disseminating stereotypes through decontextualised media spectacles.

> Through the constitution of consensual 'SM' as well as other unlegitimized 'sexualities' as objects of expert knowledge, so-called 'normal' 'heterosexuality' automatically reached the privileged position of subjectivity representing the condition of knowing. This strategical positioning of 'heterosexuality' allows it never to become an object of knowledge itself.
>
> (Beckmann, 2009, pp. 37–38)

Depression is also a category often diagnosed in women and other minoritised groups, which raises the question of the production of mental illness within the social contexts. Littlewood (1994) analysing advertisements for minor-tranquillisers and anti-depressants demonstrates how images of women are more frequent, while for other medications there is a greater presence of men. In these advertisements, women are usually portrayed as housewives or looking after children.

The consumption of psychiatric drugs has been constantly increasing worldwide (Illich, 1995; Abbing-Karahagopian et al., 2014; Olié et al., 2002, Brauer et al 2021, Marconi et al 2023, NHS 2024).

Women form the group most prescribed psychotropic drugs (Ashton, 1991) and antidepressants (Zhong et al., 2014; Olié et al., 2002). Ettorre and Riska (1995) describe an over-prescription of minor tranquillisers for the elderly, women and lower socio-economic groups, raising questions regarding structural issues related to gender, race and class. Ettorre and Riska (1995) critically analyse how gender is (not) accounted for in research, as the use of tranquillisers is seen as an emergent social problem, while it is connected to the structural inequalities which produce these problems in women (tranquilisers as social control).

Similarly, potential over-prescription for elderly people has been highlighted in studies (Bobo et al., 2019). Lopes (1999) describes the high quantity of tranquilisers and hypnotics prescribed for elderly people, and within this group, women also figure as the largest percentage of consumers both in Brazil and worldwide. Lopes (1999) notes that emotional changes are not necessarily greater in the elderly; however, people come to rely on this consumption to cope with social and individual pressures related to age. This constitutes a double movement, for while on one hand, doctors spend less time with elderly patients than with young people and prescribe more psychotropic drugs to the former group (Berger & Poirier *apud* Lopes, 1999), on the other, patients come to rely on this consumption. Moreover, the side effects of these products are greater for elderly people (Lopes, 1999).

The over-prescription of psychiatric drugs for specific groups raises a number of issues. Pressures on these groups tend to be greater, being subjected to restrictive conceptions of 'normalcy', with drugs functioning as social control. Further, the way that gender and race is understood has direct effects on how women, LGBTQI+ people, immigrants and black people are diagnosed. The operation of psychiatric diagnoses in relation to gender and sexuality, and race and age, has to be critically interrogated, while considering the suffering of the individual, the power relations that the subject is embedded in need to be accounted for. Otherwise, the risk remains of the psychiatric discourse holding the Other so constituted in a devalued social position and consequent silence. Therefore, the symptom can also reveal something about the social context.

2.2 Immigration, race and mental health: diagnosis and prescription

Debates surrounding the pathologisation and medicalisation of minoritised groups highlight the importance of situating medical knowledge and an awareness of how it can (re)produce specific social imaginaries in relation to groups that are taken as the Other in discourse. In this direction, it becomes relevant to analyse how these groups appear in public services. Returning to Phoenix's (1987) observations regarding normalised absence and pathologised presence, I highlight some aspects of this dynamic focusing on the experience of black people and immigrants in the encounter with health services, which will be further debated in the next chapter.

A number of studies have analysed how immigrants have been diagnosed in psychiatry. This has involved taking the characteristics of specific groups as characteristics of mental illness, and interpreting religious practices as symptoms of psychopathology such as those coming from African countries (Loewenthal & Cinnirella, *apud* Tosh, 2016, p. 29). As Littlewood and Lipsedge observe (1989, preface, p. 10), 'As we examined the relationship between culture and mental illness, it became clear that they were already closely related but in a rather unexpected way: the everyday life and customs of minority groups in Britain and America had been frequently characterised by politicians and doctors as pathological in themselves', rather than considering the effects of the social context into the subject.

This framing has specific effects for minoritised groups, as seen in the presence of black people in mental health institutions, who are more frequently diagnosed as schizophrenic, more frequently detained compulsorily in hospitals (together with West Indian men) (Littlewood and Lipsedge observe (1989), and more frequently admitted to forensic institutions than white people in the UK (Fernando, 2012). This is similar to the experience in the US, where black people are also more likely to be detained involuntarily in mental health hospitals, more likely to be prescribed anti-psychotic medication and less likely to be in psychotherapy (Liepsedge & Littlewood, p. 55). Liepsedge and Littlewood remind us that until 1960, black Americans and Africans were thought not to have depression, and suicide was uncommon, although it had been frequent among black slaves and Amerindians. It is vital to understand how black people and immigrants are viewed in health services, including the infantilisation of the subject viewed as childlike in the therapeutic context (Littlewood & Lipsedge, 1989).

This dynamic raises the question of the situatedness of the medical profession and psy-practices, particularly how social values are embedded in the production of mental health discourses, becoming relevant to understand Western medical perspectives. Medical institutions were established and further organised in the 17th and 18th centuries, during the European Enlightenment, carrying the values of freedom and scientific rationality, technological developments of the time and the production of modern ideals (McClintock, 1995). The centrality of colonialism for the development of modernity also has to be considered. As McClintock argues, Europeans could frame what was unfamiliar, giving a negative value to what was different, and so representing this world as deviant, undervalued and negated. How would this epistemological perspective permeate theoretical and practical developments in psychiatry? It is in this context that Fernando points out a paradox within the enlightenment project, as racism was also embedded in post-Enlightenment values, as well as expected gender norms, which operated in particular ways within this paradox of freedom and scientific reasoning. 'Major Enlightenment figures, like Hume, Kant, and Hegel, articulated unchallenged extreme racist ideas (Eze, 1997). Anti-Semitism, the Atlantic slave trade, colonialism and scientific racism, all flourished well after the ideas of freedom and dignity of the individual became widely accepted in Europe' (Fernando, 2012, p. 115). As such, the way those pre-existing ideas on race operated in the history of psychiatry and how these may permeate contemporary mental health practice requires further examination.

> In the 19th and the first part of the 20th centuries, racist theories were embedded in psychiatric knowledge – indeed in 'knowledge' in general. When, in the 18th century, arguments arose (as they still do) as to whether black people suffer more insanity than do white people, eminent psychiatrists supported the view that insanity was rare among Africans, Native Americans, and others who were in a 'savage' state –

evoking Rousseau's concept of 'noble savage'. But another stance was evident (Lewis, 1965), namely that non-Europeans were mentally degenerate because they lacked 'culture' and so incapable of showing 'mental illness' anyway. A third viewpoint voiced by American psychiatrists in the 19th century, quoting statistics of admission to asylums in different parts of the USA, was this: Black Americans were relatively free of mental illness when in slavery (in the South) but subject to mental illness once set free (in the North). Various illnesses were linked to this theory. Drapetomania, or the illness of running away (Cartwright, 1851), was one, and some psychiatrists supported slavery for black people as being conducive to their mental health almost into the 20th century. In Britain, John Langdon Down (1866) claimed that the cause of what was then called 'idiocy' – the so-called illness when people had severe learning difficulties – was a racial throwback, white people reverting to a primitive ('black') mentality. He claimed to have found that people with this diagnosis in asylums in London had physical characteristics of Malays, Ethiopians, Natives of America and Mongolians – most he said were 'Mongols'. The first psychiatric textbook to document mental illness of non-Europeans was one on adolescence by Stanley Hall (1904), founder of the American Journal of Psychology. A whole chapter was titled 'adolescent races' referring to (adult) Indians, Africans, and Native North Americans as showing the characteristics of immature white children – i.e. being psychologically underdeveloped. The (racist) under-development theme seems to continue in the discourses around psychiatry and western psychology to this day (see below). In the early part of the 20th century, Kraepelin postulated that Javanese, and by extension all Asians, did not suffer depression because they were psychologically under-developed – 'akin' (as he put it) to immature European youth (Kraepelin, 1913, 1921). This idea continued throughout the first part of the 20th century with numerous observations in Africa where the apparent lack of depression as illness was attributed to the lack of a 'sense of responsibility' (Green, 1914) and by Carothers (1953) to Africans having minds that were like those of 'leucotomized Europeans'. Carl Jung fancied himself as a specialist on black people, having visited Africa and India. After returning from a visit to the USA, he postulated his 'racial infection' theory. This was that white Americans, although belonging to the same racial stock as Europeans, had become deviant as a result of their psyches being 'pulled down' to primitive levels by living too close to black people (Jung, 1930). Since the 1939–1945 war, racism has been rejected in scientific circles and latterly in most civilised discourse in all professions However, the racist IQ movement was supported in psychology circles of the 1970s – see its critiques such as Kamin (1974) and Stott (1983) – and continues to re-appear, most recently in the work of Herrnstein and Murray (1994). Leff (1973, 1977), psychiatrist at the

> prestigious Institute of Psychiatry, analyzed cross-cultural findings that were based on traditional psychiatric research methods to conclude that Asians, Africans, and African-Americans had under-developed emotional differentiation compared to Europeans – white people. And, subtle forms of racism and what we call 'institutional racism' are far from extinct.
>
> (Fernando, 2012, pp. 115–116)

The interplay between race, gender and class in this dynamic is reflected in how mental health and health services operate, becoming crucial to interrogate how black people, immigrants, LGBTQIA+ and women experience medical and psychological practices and how this impacts psychiatric theories. In this context, the effects of colonialism (Hickling, 2020), sexism and racism (Souza, 1983) on subjectivity are undeniable, as well as its effects on the subject; additionally, it is necessary to consider how othered groups are viewed in medical theory.

Diverse forms of violence towards the Other can be noted in mental health discourse. Mills (2014, p. 86) highlights how: 'the brute and benevolent violence of development that acts with impunity, that "rescues" (Chakrabarti & Dhar, 2009); the epistemological violence of biological reductionism (Shiva, 1990); the visual violence of the "look" (Fanon, 1967/1986); and the "identity violence" of colonial and psychiatric discourse (Hook, 2005, p. 480) – and violent interpellations, where there is no "turn" ', including the violence from of mental health service delivery (such as isolation, restraint, over-prescription). Such forms of violence are situated within structural power imbalances including poverty, war and natural disaster.

An analysis of the discursive practices encompassing minoritised groups has to include an understanding of institutional and structural racism and sexism, that is, medical discourses are socially and historically situated, and as such, it is important to interrogate the effects of the (re)production of the current views on gender, race, class and sexuality in health practice (Fanon, 1986; Phoenix, 1987; Nayak & Robbins, 2019; Hook, 2004). To this end, we should consider the conception of epistemological violence elaborated by Teo (2008) in the analysis of interpretative speculations that involve minoritised and marginalised groups. Teo defines *epistemological violence* as 'an hermeneutic process (interpretative speculations of data) that has negative consequences for the "Other" ' (Teo, 2008, p. 57).

> As soon as empirical differences are interpreted (and these interpretations contain speculations), and as soon as these speculations construct the 'Other' as problematic or as inferior, with possible negative consequences for the 'Other,' one should speak of a form of violence that is produced in 'knowledge.' In these cases, interpretative speculations (and not data!) turn into *epistemological violence*.
>
> (2008, p. 57)

Teo highlights an example of this dynamic when interpretating differences in the psychological measures for IQ testing for African-Americans and European-Americans.

> Genetic speculations on the causes of Black–White differences in IQ and other mental characteristics have a long history (see Richards, 1997; Winston, 2004). Yet, there exists no genetic evidence for this hypothesis, which makes it more accurate to characterize it as a *chronic speculation*. The speculation that Blacks are genetically less intelligent than Whites is an interpretation that has negative consequences for Blacks (e.g., funding for preschool programs; expectations and attributions; school support; identity; etc.). Given the negative implications for African-Americans, and given that no genetic evidence has been established for racial differences in IQ, such speculations are not a question of bad 'taste' (see Sternberg, 2005) but a question of a *hermeneutic deficit*, which is an epistemological *and* an ethical problem.
>
> (Teo, 2008, p. 60)

In the same vein, foreigners were seen as less intelligent, in tests that did not take cultural differences into account. In the 19th century, science often asserted the natural superiority of one group over another, with racial differences often being used to describe class relations (Littlewood & Lipsedge, 1989). While the situatedness of research and the epistemological closure it encompasses is evident, this also points to a specific way that discourses on 'nature' and genetics operate, that is how discourses on race have (re)produced unequal outcomes, thereby reinforcing stereotypes. It becomes fundamental to acknowledge these interpretative differences, and whether they are accounted according to the social categories and the effect of these interpretations, and how they reproduce an epistemological violence. Moreover, an individualised view on psychiatry is embedded in these discourses, wherein distress is not understood in relation to the social context, but rather as an illness of the individual, possessing a chemically mediated treatment.

Littlewood and Lipsedge (1989) highlight these differences in relation to immigration and mental illness, and how the psychiatrist encounters the immigrant: mediated through the lens of a socially specified normality and their own personal views of minority communities. Littlewood and Lipsege highlight how these two specific groups, the mentally ill and immigrants, are significantly named as 'aliens'. The 'alien' defines the boundaries, geographic outsiders (foreigners) and the outsiders in the society (mentally ill). 'They define for him the limits of his normality by producing a boundary only inside which can he be secure' (Littlewood & Lipsedge, 1989, p. 28). The social place of the outsider, and the risk of fetishising the Other, raises the question of how psy-disciplines risk maintaining this discursive position, operating as social control, being crucial to analyse how the signifiers 'race' and 'culture'

(Giordano, 2011) operate in these encounters, and to acknowledge the cultural situatedness of the conceptualisation of mental illness and treatment, that varies across cultures.

Furthermore, how a given psychiatric perspective is applied in other contexts, thereby reproducing a decontextualised and individualised view of mental health, abstracting the subject and personifying the power relations into a mental illness, also needs to be interrogated. Mills (2014) argues that psychiatry in non-Western countries takes on a colonising character, framing people's experience in alien and alienating technical terminology and situating them as in need of care (including forced treatment and involuntary detention), which is interwoven with pharmaceutical interventions as another ground of colonisation. 'We might wonder if the pharmaceutical industry has colonized psychiatry' (Mills, 2014, p. 8).

A specific imaginary production of the Other is at play, viewed as alien, foreign, and strange(r). The Other is seen as mysterious, irrational and fascinating, instating a fetishised view of the Other. These dynamics of the encounter with Othered groups have to be seen according to the intersectional operations in play, in which a feminised imaginary of the Other is assumed, that is, seen them as child-like, dangerous, emotional and passive. The effects of these discourses on the Other are those of placing the Other in need of control/care. Mills (2014, p. 96) highlights this colonising view of the Other as being in need of guidance, often understood in terms of lack, without initiative or intellectual achievements. By contrast, they may be viewed as potentially dangerous, irrational, sexually deviant or unpredictable. These discourses are seen as constituting a specific view of the Other as archaic and old in contrast to the modern and evolved Us (McClintock, 1995). In these discursive structures, therefore, it is then necessary to interrogate the place of psychiatric practice. Based on Burman's (1994) analysis on the image of the child mobilised in charity campaigns and the 'infantilization' of the Global South, Mills points out:

> This can lead to a double bind for children of the global South, who are not only represented and conceptualized as subordinate to adults because they are children, but are doubly subordinated because they are children of the South, and arguably triply subordinated by a label of 'mental illness'. Here psychiatrization, adultism, sanism, and racism intertwine not in a sum where one is added to the other, but in a knot.
>
> (Mills, 2014, p. 97)

While the child of the South can be triply subordinated and stereotyped, this particular image can operate to infantilise the Global South more generally (Burman, 2010). The feminisation of the colonised, fetishised Other, is a relevant dimension to consider in the discursive construction of both the Other and our understanding of mental health. The child-like characteristic, among others, was analysed by Burman (2015), based on Fanon's work, highlighting the intertwined discourses within the child figure and the colonial, racial and gendered views, personifying 'the Western-generated but now globalized models of subjectivity and interiority that this installs' (Burman, 2015, p. 3).

> In this sense, childhood as a field can itself be understood as colonized (Cannella & Viruru, 2004) as well as performing a key role within colonial strategies and discourse (see e.g. Balagopalan, 2002, 2014; Stoler, 2002). Where once colonized people were explicitly positioned as child-like, now, alongside 'saving brown women from brown men', as Spivak (1988) put it, it is in the name of the child – especially the girl child, as the signifier of both deserving victimhood and site for the penetration of transnational capital (Koffman & Gill, 2013) – that imperialism is waged.
>
> (Burman, 2015, p. 3)

The dynamics of gendered and racialised views of the Other can then be seen in these various operations and how they function in health and mental health fields. It is therefore crucial when analysing the epistemology of science to incorporate the sexual and racial politics of its emergence. Hegarty (2007) highlights:

> It is becoming increasingly obvious that it is impossible to analyse the history of "scientific racism" and psychology's sexual politics as if they were separate from each other. American eugenicists, including Terman, were popular intellectuals because their political visions offered solutions to several intersecting anxieties about race, family, and gender (Kline, 2001), the ontologisation of the homosexual body was informed by scientific racism (Sommerville, 1994), discourses of homosexuality have had very uneven effects along class and race lines in the United States (e.g., Chauncey, 1994; Terry, 1999), and African Americans have often been stigmatized in social science literatures for perceived deviations from White's norms for heterosexual kinship (Cohen, 1997).
>
> (Hegarty, 2007, pp. 133–134)

For a decolonial view of mental health and the development of theoretical perspectives and medical practices that consider power relations (Hickling, 2020), the deconstruction of taken for granted social categories within the purview of mental health, as well as the inclusion of the subject's experience, knowledge and social context, is therefore paramount.

2.3 Transsexuality and homosexuality: the body and diagnosis

Psychiatric classifications are historically situated and produce a nosology of behaviour filtered through a specific phenomenology within the sphere of Western social values. Regarding the production of diagnosis, two key dynamics are notable: firstly, how psychiatric diagnoses are developed in relation to specific groups, and second, how psychiatrisation impacts these groups. In previous sub-sections, I have emphasised the effects of these dynamics on mental health diagnosis and minoritised groups. The effects and production of depression in women, for example, is seen to have an impact on our understanding of women, while it also raises questions about the social position of women. Notably, the nosography of mental health and depression combines characteristics traditionally attributed to a 'normal' woman, such as emotionality, infantility and madness (Hockey, 1993). This discursive operation can risk obliterating women's experiences and (re)produce an uncritical conception of diagnosis and medicalisation. Similarly, the epistemological violence concerning how race and the colonial background can function in psychiatric diagnosis was highlighted, particularly when interrogating the (re)production and effect of the normal and pathological distinction. In this sub-section, I will focus on the production of diagnoses markedly associated with specific groups, which will add another dimension to our reflections. Here I focus on a critical analysis of the production of 'transsexualism' and 'homosexualism' as psychiatric categories. The definition of psychiatric categories related to sexual activities and identities has been a critical point for feminist and queer theorists, who show how these diagnoses reinforce stigmatised ideas about gender and sexuality, and pathologise individuals who do not identify with specific heterosexual and gender norms.

During the 19th century, sexuality came to be psychiatrically classified in relation to normality/abnormality and a broad domain of 'perversions. Foucault (1978) argues that this view of sexuality produced a 'truth of sex', predominantly based on 'two modes of production of truth: procedures of confession, and scientific discursivity' (Foucault, 1978, pp. 64–65). In this production, contextualised moral conceptions of sex are present, placing it in a specific discursive position.

> The essential point is that sex was not only a matter of sensation and pleasure, of law and taboo, but also of truth and falsehood, that the truth of sex became something fundamental, useful, or dangerous, precious or formidable: in short, that sex was constituted as a problem of truth.
>
> (1978, p. 56)

Through techniques, procedures and rituals (of confession), the distinction between the normal and pathological is created.

> 5. through the medicalisation of the effects of confession. The obtaining of the confession and its effects were recodified as therapeutic operations. Which meant first of all that the sexual domain was no longer accounted for simply by the notions of error or sin, excess or transgres-

> sion, but was placed under the rule of the normal and the pathological (which, for that matter, were the transposition of the former categories); a characteristic sexual morbidity was defined for the first time; sex appeared as an extremely unstable pathological field: a surface of repercussion of other ailments, but also the focus of a specific nosography, that of instincts, tendencies, images, pleasure, and conduct. This implied furthermore that sex would derive its meaning and its necessity from medical interventions: it would be required by the doctor, necessary for diagnosis, and effective by nature in the cure. Spoken in time, to the proper party, and by the person who was both the bearer of it and the one responsible for it, the truth healed.
>
> (Foucault, 1979, p. 67)

Homosexuality came under psychiatric scrutiny in the 19th century, often associated with effeminacy. Despite there being no direct or causal relation between sexuality, desire and effeminacy, a number of different behaviours and identities were included in this concept, such as 'sodomy, effeminacy, gender inversion, male friendships, and same-sex relationships' (Halperin, 2000, *apud* Tosh, 2015, p. 56), having multiple and diverse histories of homosexuality. The term 'homosexuality' ('homosexualität') was coined by Kertbeny in 1869 in a leaflet challenging its criminalisation in Germany (Tosh, 2015). Homosexuality was a criminal act, under the term 'sodomy', and a 'sin against nature' for religion. From the Middle Ages, procreation was seen as the only non-sinful sexual behaviour.

These religious views on sexuality condemned several sexual acts outside of procreation (Gayle, 1984/2006; Foucault, 1978). However, it is notable that this notion of sexuality was not consistent for all religions, Tosh (2015) points out that paganism and Wicca included sexuality in their practice. Nonetheless, under colonisation, these practices came to be viewed as primitive, savage and opposed to the Christian views of civility and self-control. 'The framing of non-procreative sexuality as sinful and "animalistic" reinforced this colonial discourse of a civilized and controlled religious practice of sexuality, and distinguished it from an older religions associated with "savage" native people' (Tosh, 2015, p. 60). Federici (2017) describes the persecution of women in the Middle Ages, as heretics, comparing it to the 'theology of liberation' (p. 70). In this configuration, the heretics could be seen as a movement, denouncing social hierarchies, towards a democracy of social relations, in which women had the same rights as men (p. 83). Moreover, Tosh (2015) highlights the discursive associations between lesbians and witches in Europe from the 14th to the 17th centuries, while gay men were punished in sodomy trials until the 19th century. Ussher (1991, p. 49) referred to the term 'witch' as a 'catch-all term' applied to many women, including those who were 'openly or actively sexual' (in Tosh, 2015, p. 60).

During the 19th century, sexuality was framed in medical terms through the normality/pathology distinction. Krafft-Ebing, a key figure for this disease model through his work *Psychopathia Sexualis* of 1892, utilised the terminology of 'sexual inversion' or 'contrary sexual instinct' and defined homosexuality either as existing from birth or as an acquired sexual interest, varying according

> to the degrees of 'severity'. These were: an attraction to the same sex (degree 1); 'eviration', the development of a feminine personality (degree 2); 'metamorphis sexualis paranoica', described as when a man would feel as if they were a woman (degree 3), or they believed that they were a woman (degree 4).
>
> (Tosh, 2015, p. 62)

Homosexuality was seen as a mental disorder from 1948 under the category 'sexual deviation' (ICD-6) and as 'sociopathic personality disturbance' in 1952 by the DSM-I (American Psychiatric Association – APA). The APA in 1968 redefined it as a 'sexual deviation' in the DSM-II, and then as 'ego-dystonic homosexuality' in the DSM-III, which was later removed from the DSM-III-R (Drescher, 2015). The APA concluded that homosexuality was not a mental disorder in 1973. 'Ego-dystonic homosexuality' was removed from the DSM-III-R in 1987 (Moleiro & Pinto, 2015). The DSM IV (1994) replaced transsexualism with 'gender identity disorder in adults and adolescents'; DSM-5 (2013) replaced 'gender identity disorder' with 'gender dysphoria' (Robles et al., 2021).

The category of 'sexual deviation' appeared with the ICD-6 (WHO), as a sub-category of 'pathogenic personality', and continued in the ICD-7 (1955) and ICD-8 (1965), up until the publication of the ICD-9 (1990) which introduced the terms 'disorders of sexual preferences' and 'paraphilia', echoing the perspective developed in the DSM-III in 1980 (Giami, 2015, p. 1129). Sexual deviancy referred to behaviours such as exhibitionism, fetishism, homosexuality, pathological sexuality and sadism, and differed from 'disorders of sexual function', which were categorised as 'psychogenic reactions affecting the genito-urinary system'. These were based on the work of Krafft-Ebing (1895) and Ellis (Giami, 2015, p. 1129). The World Health Organisation removed the term in 1991. However, the definition of sexual deviations was replaced by notion of paraphilia (DSM-III, DSM-IIIR, ICD-10).

This psychiatric conception of homosexuality focused mainly on the male experience, referring to a feminised idea of homosexuality, and understands gender non-conformity as an extension of homosexuality, as transgender identity was seen as more 'severe' and a 'delusion (Tosh, 2016). Both homosexuality and the transgender experience were viewed as pathologies, under the category 'perversion'. This psychiatric diagnosis continues under the term 'paraphilia', meaning 'abnormal' 'love' (Tosh, 2015). 'In addition to the already described "metamorphosis sexualis paranoica", cross-dressing and gender nonconformity have been controversially associated with several diagnoses related to sexuality, including the highly contested "transvestism" and "autogynephilia"' (Tosh, 2016, p. 51).

The term transsexuality was first used by Magnus Hirschfeld (1868–1935), a homosexual Jewish German physician who differentiated sexual orientation (at that time called 'desire orientation') from gender identity (Rodrigues et al., 2021, p. 2). Hirschfeld founded the Institute for Sexual Science in Berlin in 1919, where he performed the first sex change surgeries in the 1920s. In 1930, sex reassignment surgery was performed on Lili Elbe at the Institute. In 1933 Hitler closed the Institute and destroyed the archive (2021, p. 2).

'Transsexualism' and 'gender disorder' were introduced in the 1980s as psychiatric categories, applied to people whose identity did not match their assigned gender. Transgenderism relates to people whose gender identity does not match the assigned gender, or physically or socially established gender norms (Tosh, 2015).

The DSM-1 and DSM-2 placed 'transvestism' under the deviations of sexuality section (APA, 1952, 1968). The DSM-3 used the term 'paraphilia' and listed 'transvestism' in this category. Different to the diagnosis of 'fetishism' as based on the sole focus of women's clothing (APA, 1980), transvestism refers to wearing female clothing (completely or partially) and the participation in the transvestic subculture (Tosh, 2015).

Tosh (2015) critically analyses the inclusion of 'gender identity disorder' in the DSM III given that this diagnosis could be used for 'feminine boys' and transgender individuals, thereby intertwining pathologising history of homosexuality and gender nonconforming femininity. 'Numerous terms have been applied to a wide range of gender nonconformists, some who may identify as transgender while others may not. These include "transvestism" (APA, 1952, 2000), "transsexualism" (APA, 1980), "autogynephilia" (APA, 2013), "psychic hermaphrodism" (Krafft-Ebing, 1895), the more recent "gender dysphoria" (APA, 2013), and many more' (Tosh, 2015, p. 77).

Moreover, strong criticisms since the inclusion of 'transvestism' in the 'sexual deviation' section in the DSM-I have been voiced against the association between crossdressing and 'deviance' (Tosh, 2015). Nonetheless, the association between eroticism and sexual deviance remained with the categories 'transvestic fetishism' in 1980 (APA, 1980) and subsequently 'transvestic disorder with/without fetishism' (APA, 2013). In the DSM-3, additional descriptions were included, and in the DSM-5, this association was strengthened with the term 'autogynephilia' in the 'transvestic disorder' diagnostic criteria, defined as 'males [who are] erotically aroused by the thought or image of themselves as women' (Blanchard, *apud* Tosh, 2015, pp. 81–82). This diagnosis has been criticised due to its eroticisation and to the amount of cisgender women who satisfied these criteria. Tosh (2015) continues describing how the absence of autoandrophilia from the DSM-5 could also show the psychiatric interest in gender noncomforming femininty. 'The pathologization of gender nonconformity is divided into a fetishized behaviour (cross-dressing) and an identity "disorder" (transgender or non-binary identities)' (Tosh, 2016, p. 47). The pathologisation of gender non-conforming people is seen in the replacement of diagnosis, showing how the conception of a causal relationship between sex, gender identity and sexuality (desire, practice) operates in these perspectives.

The current DSM-5 includes intersexuality and defines 'gender dysphoria' (with/without a sex development disorder), formulated as 'a marked incongruence between one's experienced/expressed gender and assigned gender' (APA, 2013, p. 452 in Tosh, 2015, p. 87). It is interesting to note the elements seen as symptoms, which also reveals specific expectations according to gender and sexuality, such as 'in boys, a strong rejection of typically masculine toys, games, and activities and a strong avoidance of rough-and-tumble play; in girls, a strong rejection of typically feminine toys, games, and activities' (p. 452 in Tosh, 2015, p. 93).

In the ICD-10 (WHO), the diagnosis appears in Chapter V, relating to 'Mental and behavioural disorders', and appears as transsexualism:

> [a] desire to live and be accepted as a member of the opposite sex, usually accompanied by a sense of discomfort with, or inappropriateness of, one's anatomical sex, and a wish to undergo surgery and hormonal treatment to make one's body as congruent as possible with one's preferred sex.
>
> (in Martinez-Guzman et al., 2014, p. 9)

The World Health Organisation removed 'sexual identity disorder' (more specifically termed 'transsexualism') from the disease-related chapter of the ICD and relocated it as 'gender incongruence' into another chapter associated with 'other conditions related to sexual health' (WHO, 2019). For the ICD-11, transsexuality is designated as 'gender incongruence' (Rodrigues Carneiro & Nogueira, 2021, p. 4), which is a change from a pathologising view of gender nonconforming people. The World Health Organisation defines it as:

> ICD-11 has redefined gender identity-related health, replacing diagnostic categories like ICD-10's 'transsexualism' and 'gender identity disorder of children' with 'gender incongruence of adolescence and adulthood' and 'gender incongruence of childhood', respectively. Gender incongruence has thus broadly been moved out of the 'Mental and behavioural disorders' chapter and into the new 'Conditions related to sexual health' chapter. *This reflects evidence that trans-related and gender diverse identities are not conditions of mental ill health*, and classifying them as such can cause enormous stigma. Inclusion of gender

> incongruence in the ICD should ensure transgender people's access to gender-affirming health care, as well as adequate health insurance coverage for such services. Recognition in the ICD also acknowledges the links between gender identity, sexual behaviour, exposure to violence and sexually transmitted infections.[3]

These psychiatric diagnostics produced the basis for a number of medical interventions, including prevention of 'transsexualism' in children, with the diagnosis of 'gender identity disorder in childhood', now under the category of 'gender dysphoria in children'. The diagnosis based on gender dysphoria in children and its corrective treatment was challenged by 'affirming' programmes which view gender non-conformity as a healthy human expression (Pyne, 2014).

There is already a long trajectory of debates on the effects of the pathologisation of individuals, and the understanding of transsexuality as a psychiatric disorder, which was contested by trans activists (e.g. Stop Transpathologisation Campaign) and academics (Missé & Coll-Planas, 2011; Arán e Murta, 2009). Nonetheless, in some countries, there is a debate on the need to maintain this categorisation for access to medical support and intervention; for this, there is a pressure to remove the psychiatric diagnosis but continue the guarantee of medical support. Rodrigues et al. (2021, p. 9) argue that when a trans person can only access health services under the label trans, there is a need to perform as such, 'become absolutely "obedient" to a system that has the power to try to normalize their bodies and identities. When people become disobedient, access to health is blocked, creating paths of increased oppression for these people'. Some trans activists and researchers have proposed a change of direction that moves from the 'paradigm of disorder' to the 'paradigm of diversity' (Missé & Coll-Planas, 2010 *apud* Martinez-Guzman et al., 2014, p. 13).

The forms of pathologisation, diagnosis and treatment within psy-disciplines have been criticised due to the resulting increased stigma and control over trans people (Martinez-Guzman et al., 2014). The effects of these dichotomic definitions have been extensively contested (Missé & Coll-Planas, 2011; Tosh, 2015), as they risk further marginalising these minoritised groups and provide only limited discursive space for alternative sexual expressions. This medical framework can also function by implying that all trans people seek the same bodily changes (Suess, 2011). These classifications view transsexualities as a problem of the individual and displace the effect of transphobia onto the subject. 'The individual is responsible for sex-gender non-conformity, and not society for transphobia' (Arán; Zaidhaft; Murta, 2008 apud Rodrigues et al., 2021, p. 4), Ansara and Hegarty (2011) similarly argue in their study of the psychological pathologisation of children and the effects of cisgenderism on the subject.

The process of declassifying homosexuality as a mental illness was initiated in the 1980s. In Brazil, it was only in 1999 that homosexuality ceased to be seen as a mental disorder by the Psychology Council (Conselho Federal de Psicologia), although there is still pressure from conservative religious psychologists to allow forms of conversion therapy. While conversion therapy is a name for a range of methods, some professionals avoid using the term due to its negative connotations and professional regulations. In the other contexts, psychiatric interest turned to the 'pre-homosexual child', particularly effeminate or 'feminine boys' (Tosh, 2016). 'Rekers used behavioural therapy such as advising parents to reward masculine behaviour and punish feminine behaviours. This included high levels of monitoring, with professionals and parents observing the child's behaviour intensely and providing a response depending on their play, dress, or actions' (Pyne, 2014). Punishments included physical discipline (e.g. 'swatting') by parents, in some cases (Rekers, 1977). Further concerns and criticisms of conversion therapies applied on children have been expressed (Pyne, 2014), also regarding the long-term effects.

Increased suicide rates as a result of 'conversion therapy' have been widely documented (see Tosh, 2016). Furthermore, the effect of transphobia on suicide rates and suicide attempts (Clements-Nolle et al., 2006) within trans communities has to be fully considered, having long been an area of concern (around 40% of trans people try to end their life prior to receiving medical support, rising to 60% when medical care is refused (Tosh, 2016, p. 64)), as well as the risk of violence against trans people (e.g. the high number of homicides in Brazil). Therapies that affirm the subject's gender identity were seen to reduce the risk of suicide, 'mostly when families support the individuals in some cases suicide attempts have been reduced by 93 per cent' (Travers et al., 2012 *apud* Tosh, 2016, p. 48).

This raises several key issues regarding the reproduction of moral conceptions of gender and sexuality within psychiatry and psychology. Therefore, it is vital for practice to consider the social context and structural transphobia, which I will further consider in Chapter 4. Understanding the effects of transphobia on the experience of trans people is vital (Coll-Planas, 2011), in addition to understanding the development of coping strategies (Platero Méndez, 2014). *Stop Trans Pathologization* 2012, organised by the International Trans Depathologization Network, aims to remove gender identity disorder from the DSM and the IDC, as well as doing away with the need for a mandatory psychiatric diagnosis for hormonal and surgical treatments and for changing name and sex on the civil registry (Rodrigues et al., 2021). There has been a call for the right to full participation by trans people in decisions regarding access to hormonal and surgical treatments, which as Suess (2011) has argued, produces a juridical regime of recognition rather than one of authorisation. In this sense, the conceptualisation of trans-knowledge of Martinez-Guzman et al. (2014, p. 16) becomes relevant:

> Trans-knowledge seeks to give rise to paradoxical and ambivalent readings that question the dominant order of sex/gender and celebrate alternative practices, at the same time that they are sensitive to the

> multiplicity of experiences and perspectives of those who incorporate these practices. Trans-knowledge does not reject the use of identity categories, but it does not hide behind them. It does not seek to solidify perspectives, nor to bring identity positions to a closure, but to keep both open to the possibility of transformation hoping to generate increasingly inclusive social conditions.

Currently the diversity in the trans community is expressed through the differences between local definitions of transgender and the intersections between race, sexuality, class, age and disability. The definitions of trans people can be seen broadly as *Travesti*, Transgender and Transsexual, among other regional definitions. ANTRA (Associação Nacional de Travestis e Transsexuais, Brazilian Travesti and Transsexual Association) highlights that several activist groups in the latest Brazilian National LGBTQI+ conference defined the T for LGBTQIA+ as standing for: *Travestis*, transwomen, transmen and transmasculine people. *Travesti* refers to a typically Latin American identity with a greater presence in Brazil and Argentina. 'Frequently, *travesti* transcends binarism and moves between genders. Despite their predominantly female gender expression, they break with masculine and feminine, constructing another possible body by broadening the spectrum of femininity'.[4]

2.4 The production of drug addiction and minoritised groups

The history of the formulation of the psychiatric classification of drug addiction is grounded in the intertwined dynamics of medicine, law and religion. Compulsive behaviour related to drug use, as well as other compulsive behaviours, came to be seen as a mental illness in the 20th century. The way that discourses on drugs have impacted groups such as the working class (Berridge & Edwards, 1987), immigrants (Kohn, 1992), Black people (MacRae, 2016a), homosexuals (Keire, 1998) and women (Campbell, 2000) will be further analysed here.

Conceptions about drugs and drug use are saturated by a specific moral framework. While debates regarding their understanding highlight the lack of a clear definition of drugs, drug use and addiction, this has not hindered the creation and implementation of a number medical interventions and juridical applications. The current definition of drugs varies according to medical, juridical and religious conceptions. As a social function, drugs are seen as food, medicine and poison, used in recreational ways, in medical practices, as a social habit and in religious rituals (Xiberras, 1989; Escohotado, 1998; McKenna, 1992; Goodman et al., 1995; South, 1999; MacRae, 1998; Courtwright, 1995; Varella, 2013; Fernandes, 2011).

Within the religious sphere, and more specifically for most Christian traditions, when used in a recreational way, drugs are seen as evil substances, symbolising impurity. When used in religious rituals, however, such as sacramental wine, they are viewed as 'sacred' or 'Christ's blood'. In other religious contexts, such as the use of ayahuasca in Brazilian Santo Daime rituals, it is also seen as sacred 'Christ's blood' or 'divine being' (MacRae, 2016a), as a 'plant of power'.

From a medical perspective, a commonly used definition for drugs would be any exogenous chemical substance that provokes functional and/or structural effects (Mountian, 2013a). Drugs refer to all the substances, either legal or illegal, that cause physical alterations. The World Health Organisation (WHO) classifies drugs as:

> In the context of international drug control, 'drug' means any of the substances in Schedule I and II of the 1961 Convention, whether natural or synthetic. A term of varied usage. In medicine, it refers to any substance with the potential to prevent or cure disease or enhance physical or mental welfare; in pharmacology it means any chemical agent that alters the biochemical or physiological processes of tissues or organisms.
>
> (United Nations Office for Drug Control and Drug Prevention, 2016, p. 63)

This view of drugs based on medical and legal regulations is seen as a mark for the contemporary conception of drugs. This classification, however, does not provide a clear definition, as a too wide range of substances are classified as drugs, without a chemical unity, or similar effects. Despite this lack of clear definition (South, 1999; McMurran, 1994; Loose, 2002a, 2002b), discourses about addiction are often applied to the use of specific drugs, most frequently to illegal substances and legal ones when not used for medical or religious purposes.

The juridical classification of drugs, defining those that are legal and illegal, had a major impact into the way that drugs are understood and utilised. Arnao (2002) argues that the scientific word narcotic[5] became a legal-bureaucratic term that defines these substances according to their legal status. 'The word "narcotics" had been purged of its scientific meaning and became, instead, a symbol of socially disapproved drugs' (2002, p.1). The issue of the definition of drugs has been a central debate for scientific and legal thought. Escohotado (1998, vol. 1, p. 21) points out: 'The international authority for public health declared that the problem is insoluble because of its extra-pharmacological spheres, thus proposing to classify drugs as legal and illegal' (1998, vol. 1, p. 21).

The question of addiction raises similar issues, remaining ambiguous and paradoxical, with commentators arguing that drug addiction has become a matter of convention, rather than of pharmacological definition (Bucher, 1992; Szasz, 1975). Definitions of drugs and drug addiction are intrinsically related to the social and moral values imbued in them. 'The substance is always the cultural values invested in it, and this applies whether the values be those of the police, the pharmacologist or the user' (McDonald, 1994, p. 19).

Therefore, the definition of drugs appears fluid making room for various interpretations with specific discursive effects. Thus, as mere things (entities) they only have meaning when they are in order-to (Heidegger, 1997), they possess a function and manipulability that confers their characteristics and, at the same time, refers to the subject who manipulates them in specific contexts. In the same vein, Vargas (2008) drawing on Deleuze and Guattari (1997) refers to drugs as socio-technical objects, which are those objects that remain indeterminate until reported to those agencies that constitute them as such.

In this sense, the term *pharmakon*, from the Greek, meaning both medicine and poison, can provide further insight, as it reveals simultaneously good and evil qualities. Derrida (1997) highlights that pharmakon (writing) this 'medicine', this filter, that is at the same time remedy and poison, is introduced to the body of discourse with all its ambivalence. It carries a quality of fascination and power of enchantment, which oscillates ambiguously between good and evil. The *pharmakon* has no stable essence or identity, or unique character, nor is it a substance (metaphysical, physical, chemical or alchemical) in any sense of the word. This non-identity, nonessence, nonsubstance thought within a philosophical perspective gives us some insight into the complexity or ambivalence of the process when searching for an adequate definition for the notion of drugs.

Drug discourse foundations: medicine, law and religion

The use of psychoactive plants can be observed in nearly all societies (McKenna, 1992; Escohotado, 1998; Douglas, 1987; Goodman et al., 1995), except for communities in Arctic zones, where the climate does not provide the conditions for vegetation (Escohotado, 1998). The first written record of such plants was opium use by the Sumerians in 5000 BC (Szasz, 1975; Escohotado, 1998). The use of psychoactive substances is a plural phenomenon, which changes according to the time, place and purpose for use, be it therapeutic, religious, medical or habitual.

The role of the law can be seen as decisive in the contemporary understanding of drugs. Xiberras (1989) highlights that the traditional use of drugs, such as alcohol consumption in the occident and cannabis in the orient, did not cause rejection, being part of accepted social practice, different to the modern context of the last two centuries, where legal censure came to characterise drug use. A number of authors highlight how the term 'drug' has become associated with prohibition (Ruggiero, 1999), having important effects on the (in)visibility of illegal drug use.

Escohotado (1998, vol. 2) proposes five main arguments for the context of prohibition and drug control: the traditional religious element (impurity); social tensions in relation to the working class and industrialisation (drugs symbolising the deviancy of certain groups – Chinese, Mexican, black people); the evolution of the medical profession (like the ecclesiastics of other times);

the state assuming functions that were previously performed by civil society (Welfare State); and the Chinese-English conflict (highlighting stereotypes and colonial relations). I will also include gender and sexuality as another key aspect (e.g. fear of inter-racial marriage, social control).

Another major shift in the understanding of drugs was the view of drug addiction as a disease, becoming the main paradigm for medical practice, research, legal categorisation and popular discourse. An analysis of underlying moral values provides an important basis to understand the contemporary notion of addiction. For this, I emphasise some aspects of North American and English drug policies, which had a far-reaching impact on drug policies worldwide.

In the 18th and 19th centuries, alcohol consumption came to be viewed in the US and the UK as problematic, due to its increasing consumption and the new social relations resulting from industrialisation. In this context, McDonald (1994) highlights how 'alcohol turned into a serious threat to the economic and moral order. Abstinence was then equivalent to respect, self-control, hard work and thrift, all qualities indicative of religious commitment and economic prosperity'. A healthy person meant abstaining from alcohol and having a good, pure and well-ordered existence. This conception of health, which contributed to the subsequent formulation of addiction as a disease, requires social and cultural contextualisation. Developed in Britain and the U.S., this approach was highly influenced by positivism, which sought to explain behaviour based on methods of natural science. The underlying idea of addiction as a disease of the will, then simply as a disease, led both countries to understand addiction as associated with criminality, underground sub-cultures, demanding a consequent emphasis on control and prohibition (Zieger, 2008).

It is noteworthy that religious movements had an impact on fields that were viewed as morally deviant, such as sexuality (e.g. homosexuality) and inebriety, previously known as 'habitual drunkenness', which came to be understood as a 'disease' (McDonald, 1994, p. 2). Inebriety was a term used for several drugs, gaining prominence in the late 19th century through former Temperance activists physicians (Zieger, 2008). It fell out of use, however, in the mid-20s to be replaced by alcoholism, addiction or dependency (White, 2004).

In the US, the notion of addiction was initially related to Protestant notions of self-control, where drug addicts were seen as having a 'disease of the will'. In Britain, also for the Temperance movement – influential during the 19th and 20th centuries – there was a belief in the sinfulness and degradation of those who consumed alcohol (Gusfield, 1997). The Temperance movement had its origins in the 1820s, with the American Temperance Society being formed in 1826. The Liverpool Temperance Society was founded in 1830 while the moderation society in Scotland began in 1828 (Harrison, 1971). The British and Foreign Temperance Society was a London-based reform society following the traditional evangelical model with Quakers and women playing a prominent role. Temperance ideas viewed alcohol as particularly dangerous: 'the moral, religious, political and legal spotlights turned alcohol in such a way that it appeared, of itself, capable of producing social effects of all kinds' (McDonald, 1994, p. 3). Advocating for abstinence, drunkenness was considered a sin. As an evil substance *per se*, alcohol was seen as the source of addiction.

In the 19th century, ideas about opium also began to change, going from a rather accepted use, for medical and semi-medical purposes, to a view of disease and social disapproval (Berridge, 1989). The Pharmacy Act in 1868 controlled opium use, although restrictions were still minimal and prescriptions with opium were still available (Berridge & Edwards, 1987). Opium was consumed by all levels of society, mostly as a domestic medicine for all sorts of minor complaints, including excessive drinking, although historically more attention has been given to recreational opium use. In general, opium use was not viewed as a 'problem', and users were not seen as ill or addicted. As Dally (1996, p. 203) argues 'addicts, formerly objects of mild disapproval, rather like drunks or smokers today, were gradually turned into criminals and outcasts'.

Berridge and Edwards (1987) describe this change of public perception of opium. From the recreational use by romantic poets (upper classes), which attracted media attention, to the middle- and working-class self-medication and social consumption, to the conception of addiction as a disease. In late 1830s, doctors became involved in controlling opium use, 'From being one among many prescribers of the drug, with nothing approaching unitary control, they began to re-define opium use as solely a medical imprint, it became a disease, a habit warranting medical intervention. Doctors became the custodian of a problem which they had helped define' (Berridge & Edwards, 1987, p. 76).

This movement from the 1850s and 1860s that sought to end or reduce opium use was important for the establishment of the medical profession, and the origins of psychiatry, as well as for governmental support for medicine and the emergence of a drug centred approach, remains the backbone of contemporary drug policy. Berridge and Edwards (1987, p. 78) argue that 'concentration on simple statistical results without an awareness of social context or economic reality produced a situation which justified the restriction of open sale of the drug. Opium, as elsewhere, was the scapegoat for broader defects in the society of the time'.

Studies into opium use were also the basis for the disease theory of addiction. Treatment involved physical methods such as the Galvanic method (electric shock) in the 1840s, until the end of the century (Berridge & Edwards, 1987). Another area of concern was 'morphinism', despite little evidence of large numbers of morphine addicts and no sub-culture. Morphinism was defined by Dr Levinstein (in Berlin) in 1877 as a disease similar to dipsomania, but not a mental disease. There was an association between morphinism and women during the 1880s, who were seen as more susceptible than men, although there were more male consumers (1987). Women were medicated with opium for a number of female issues (e.g. childbirth, menstrual pain, etc.) and for the gender biased notions of 'nervous disorder' and hysteria. Morphine was viewed as a prescription for women for 'bourgeois femininity' (Keire, 1998, p. 809). In the US, most medical addicts were women, and addiction was seen as feminine (Keire, 1998). Furthermore, 'alcoholism', a term coined for chronic intoxication by the Swedish physician Magnus Huss in 1849 (White, 2004), was viewed as a disease during this period (Berridge & Edwards, 1987). The term 'alcoholism' came to be used in the mid-20th century, despite controversies regarding the precision of the term, for example, in 1941 Jellinek proposed fourteen types of problematic alcohol consumption (White, 2004).

By 1900, medicine was even more organised, institutionalised and developed (e.g. immunisation, bacterial research) (Acker, 1996, p. 115). In this period, there was also another shift in the understanding of psychotropic drugs, from one drug to tackle a range of illnesses to specific drugs targeting specific illnesses (Moncrieff, 2008). Opium, in this sense, was a central concern, losing its place in popular culture and medical practice. While self-medication was on the decline, the British working-class continued to use opium (*laudanum*), such as in the baby's bottle (Berridge & Edwards, 1987). The disease theory became central for contemporary drug discourses. Berridge and Edwards (1987, p. 229) argue:

> The disease view of addiction with its implicit notions of constitutional or hereditary predisposition established an individualistic, privatising ideology, nominally value-free. Medical concepts reinforced and reflected existing social structures. A distinct area of ideological terrain had been won.

By the beginning of the 20th century in the USA, medicine conceived addiction as a bio-psychological condition. The physiological model was centred on the substance, which would induce addiction, and for the psychological perspective, the focus was on the psychology of the user, where it was believed that pre-existing psychological elements (inherent neurosis, congenital manic-depression) would make people susceptible to drug addiction. 'The contemporary support for eugenics, as well as the concern with psychopathic criminality among scholars and criminal justice professionals provided a very conducive atmosphere to these theories' (Ghatak, 2010, p. 48). It is crucial to highlight that in both models, there was no attempt made to understand drugs within their social context.

It is important to distinguish this 19th-century understanding, from current perspectives on drug use, addiction and health. The three main discursive foundations on drug use – the religious influence (evangelical and temperance movements), growing status of the medical profession (expansion of psychiatry) and state regulation – were seen to provide the basis for contemporary discourses about drugs, which have a crucial impact into the groups that are positioned as the Other.

Aspects on gender, race, class and sexuality in the history of drugs

The view of drugs as a great threat became predominant throughout the 20th century, particularly after the First World War, when specific associations started to emerge connecting drug use, ethnic minorities, the working class, women and LGBTQI people. As Zieger (2008, p. 9) highlights, the British and North American 'cultural histories of addiction both form around a mobile concept of colonial seduction leading inexorably to a debilitating imperial dependency and compulsion'. This is based on ideas of addiction as being close to slavery, in opposition to modern and enlightened conceptions of agency.

The way that gender, sexuality, race and class were mobilised in this context is crucial to understand how drug policy was developed and operates for specific groups. Examples can be seen in discourses about the fear of race mixing grounded in the 'vulnerability of white women' and the 'dangerousness accorded to black men'. In this context, drug use by white people was seen as an 'individual aberration', different to black and working-class individuals. Drugs were viewed as a cult activity, with women being the most at risk of drug habit and sexual immorality.

After the First World War, a xenophobic climate was prevalent, which can be seen in perspectives grounded in a complex of 'vice, race, corruption and drugs' (South, 1994, p. 2). Alcohol came to be seen as a social problem, due to the influence of the Temperance movement: '"We are fighting Germans, Austrians and Drink, and so far as I can see, the greatest of these deadly foes is Drink", Lloyd George declared in 1915' (Kohn, 1992, p. 28). In England, this was seen for example in the closure of pubs in the afternoon, until 1988. In 1915, there was the midnight curfew at weekends for clubs, while restaurants and pubs could serve food only until nine-thirty p.m. Kohn (1992) argues that this created the conditions for the emergence of illegal night-clubs that went underground. During the Great War in Britain, women started to occupy working positions and seen in public. This public presence was highly sexualised: 'a "public woman" was a prostitute' (Kohn, 1992, p. 52).

This transition period, characterised by social changes, including to women's status, carried paternalistic and xenophobic overtones that reflected in drug policies, such as a fear of race mixing and the assumption of women's 'atavistic passions' induced by alcohol and drugs. The Chinese and Jamaicans played the role of villain within drug discourses during this period (Kohn, 1992). In the UK and US, for example, there was a panic surrounding the relationship between white women and Chinese men due to opium use and gambling (*pai-ke-p'iao*), with women being seen as the primary victims. The *Empire News* referred to the Chinese as the 'moral yellow peril' (Kohn, 1992). Opium was banned in the U.S. in 1909, generating significant effects on the Chinese community, leading to spectacularised deportations. Musto (1999) argues that the prohibition of smoking opium was also used as a symbolic marker in the U.S. fight against the evils of addiction.

Although in the U.S., the association between Chinese immigrants and opium use was well established, most of the new visible 'addicts' were in fact neither Chinese or opium smokers (Hickman, 2000). However, Hickman argues that 'fear of the Chinese and the black shaped American drug policy. This world of Oriental otherness thus threatened the stability of the bourgeois subject – while also defining it' (Hickman, 2000, p. 71).

> Early-twentieth-century drug discourse linked the age of dope to the practices of the 'oriental' through the figure of the 'white slaver'. The primitivised subcultural styles and sites of jazz clubs and dance halls, and the domestic and leisure activities of the working classes, recent immigrants, and African-American communities were also associated with the drug threat. The primitivising rhetoric applied to the lower and working classes; the orientalising register applied to the self-indulgence of the upper and middle classes – native-born women supplied by unscrupulous physicians, traffickers in women, and 'oriental drug smugglers'.
>
> (Campbell, 2000, p. 61)

In England and the United States, as well as in other Western countries, discourses focused on three main discursive dynamics and their intersections: the primitivised (working class, immigrant), the orientalised (upper class use), and the sexualised (gender and sexuality) imaginary. Since the 19th and the beginning of the 20th centuries, addicts were frequently identified with foreign groups and internal minorities, against a backdrop of an increasingly forceful national identity. These groups were already feared and the object of elaborate and far-reaching (both social and legal) constraints. The two main oppressed groups associated with drug use were the Chinese (opium) (Zinberg, 1984) and black people (cocaine) (Dally, 1996). Reports also began to appear linking cocaine and crime (also of sexual nature). As Zieger (2008, p. 242) highlights, the invention of the addict draws on polarised discursive positions of the 'master and slave, consumer and producer, men and women, straight and queer, white and race, citizen and pathological criminal'.

In the US by the start of the 20th century, 'cocaine was said to destroy the moral senses, turning women into prostitutes, boys into thieves and men into hardened killers' (Courtwright, 1995, p. 10). Among these sensationalist images, there were also associations between cocaine use and homosexuality (Keire, 1998).

The association with homosexuality, for example, could be observed at the meeting of the American Psychiatric Association in 1934. Marihuana was regarded as

> a primary stimulus to the impulsive life with direct expression in the motor field. [It] releases inhibitions and restraints imposed by society and allows individuals to act out their drives openly [and] act as sexual stimulant [particularly to] overt homosexuals.
>
> (Musto, 1999, p. 220)

In 1978, in the *Congresso Latino-Americano de Farmacologia*, a book was distributed called *Marihuana – yerba maldita* (marihuana – malevolent herb), connecting homosexuality and marihuana use (Masur & Carlini, 1994, p. 85).

Addiction was seen as a kind of bondage 'modelled on slavery that affected whites' (Campbell, 2000, p. 72), producing fear and justifying punitive methods against addicts and suppliers. The mobilisation of fear in drug discourses played a crucial role. In the 1920s fear of cannabis was beginning to emerge, although the use was still minimal throughout the U.S., associated with the Mexicans, associating crime and marihuana (Musto, 1999). MacRae (2016) highlights that in Brazil, cannabis (*ganja*) used for medical, religious, recreational and cultural purposes has been linked to people coming from Africa and indigenous people since colonisation. Brazilian authorities banned its sale in 1932.

In the U.S., recreational alcohol consumption was prohibited (1920–1933), driving the expansion of an illegal alcohol market and increasing health risks (Royal College of Psychiatrists, 2000; Rodrigues, 2003). Alcoholics Anonymous was founded in 1930s.

After the Second World War, with a period of advances in pharmaceutical technologies and drug development (e.g. antibiotics, vaccines, birth control pills and psychotropic drugs), there was a change in understanding surrounding psychotropic drugs, as anti-psychotics and anti-depressants came onto the market as consumer goods – 'happy pills' (Herzberg, 2009), based on the idea of specific drugs for specific purposes (e.g. treating abnormal brain states) contrasting with the earlier drug model of drugs inducing abnormal states through sedation or stimulation (Moncrieff, 2008).

Although several studies (see Moncrieff, 2008; Healy, 2004) contest the widespread psychiatric diagnosis: the way that depression has been diagnosed, the over-prescription of psychiatric drugs, inaccuracy of scientific research, drug trials in the case of depression (and other diagnosis) and the relations between pharmaceutical companies and medical practice (Healy, 2004; Goldberg, 1999), this model is still central to contemporary psychiatry and medicine. Further, the category stimulants was changed to 'anti-depressants' in 1963, and in 1980, depression was included in the DSM III as mental illness. Moncrieff (2008, p. 2352) highlights that the 'concept of the antidepressant helped to fashion our modern notion of depression'.

In the USA within the context of the Second World War, further 'foreign' associations were made, with the fear that the Japanese could smuggle opium into the US, suggesting a 'new form of chemical warfare' (Campbell, 2000, p. 64). Later in the 1950s and 60s, the drug threat extended to Russia, Asia and China: 'communism menaced modern democracy with "brainwashing" or "Pavlovian mind control" achieved through drugs. These constructions position the US as a "victim nation", despite its high rate of drug consumption, becoming a key actor in drug restrictions worldwide' (Campbell, 2000).

Prevalent cultural images connecting women to drugs, promoted two polarised imaginaries: the victim and the threat. While the addicted white woman was an 'exotic' character, the opium vampire embodied the polarised opposite of the woman's child-like innocence. Hence, the image of the vampire contrasts with that of the addict who flirts with death (Zieger, 2008). Through stories that addiction could spread, and the danger presented to women, the Chinese became a threat to family and society. These ideas were popularised in books (e.g. *Opium: The Demon Flower*, 1926 (Campbell, 2000)) and in exploitation movies (Mountian, 2013a).

> Drug policy provides a case study of the interplay between political power, knowledge production, and a parade of fantastic figures – the 'morphinist mothers' and 'opium vampires' of the nineteenth and early twentieth centuries, the 'enemies within' and the 'girl drug addict' of the 1950s, the 'heroin mothers' of the 1970s, and the 'crack moms' of more recent memory.
>
> (Campbell, 2000, p. 12)

This social imaginary related to drugs and drug users was disseminated in the US, creating the possibility for political pressure on overarching policies adopted worldwide. During the 20th century, several drug regulations were enacted, culminating in the prohibition of a series of drugs in 1961 and a further amendment in 1972[6] (Rodrigues, 2003). While religious discourses prevailed during the 19th century, in the 20th, we witnessed their replacement by medicalised discourses and state regulations (Stimson, 1994, p. 314).

Contemporary drug policies: an overview

Drug policies are designed and implemented according to social values, political perspectives and public opinion. These often oscillate between punitive and therapeutic approaches, with specific outcomes for groups according to gender, race, class, age, sexuality and drug type. The UN international guidelines are implemented and adapted for each context (Rodrigues, 2003; Machado & Miranda, 2007).

The changes that occurred in the 20th century were decisive for drug legislation, policy and treatment. In the 1960s, campaigns targeted youths, particularly for marihuana, often employing sensationalist material. Another group that was targeted was the working class (Dally, 1996).

In the US, Nixon declared the 'war on drugs' in 1972, with far-reaching consequences for countries that were considered 'producers' (Rodrigues, 2003). Alcohol and tobacco were not on the list, as these were considered part of American cultural habits (Musto, 1999). During the Carter government (late 1970s), a more tolerant approach was adopted, with treatment being promoted rather than incarceration. It was argued that 'penalties against possession of a drug should not be more damaging to an individual than the use of the drug itself; and where they are, they should be changed' (Musto, 1999, p. 261). During the Reagan administration (1980s), policy returned to an intolerant, more hard-line approach, emphasising a reduction in availability, a 'national crusade against drugs' with the motto 'just say no' and drug tests being implemented in workplaces. During the Bush administration, drug policies adopted a 'zero tolerance' approach, including for alcohol and officially declaring a 'war on drugs'. Pressure was placed on Latin American and other countries to stop coca growing (Musto, 1999). Intolerance of drugs was widespread, as well as connections with minorities, affecting the incarceration rates for specific groups, such as having more black than white offenders for crack-cocaine (Musto, 1999). Dorn and Lee (1999) argue that the groups most likely to receive aggressive enforcement are minorities (African Americans, Hispanics), as well as low-income citizens with little education. During the Clinton government, the mandatory minimum sentence for crack and cocaine was reviewed, being 25–75 grams for crack and 125–375 grams for cocaine.

In the 1980s, in the UK, heroin was portrayed as a drug for white and Asian people, while African-Caribbean people were more associated with cannabis and crack-cocaine, stereotypically linking it with violence, 'loose living', poor education, poverty and single motherhood. Further, Murji (1999) argues that the association with marihuana gave the police excessive powers to search young Black men.

In the early 1990s, harm reduction approaches were further developed in the UK, the Netherlands and the US, primarily seeking to reduce HIV[7] among intravenous users. In contrast to abstinence policies, harm reduction aims to decrease or prevent drug use, or reduce harm resulting from drug use. It is based on pragmatism, human rights, public health and dialogue, considering drug users as part of the wider community (Inciardi & Harrison, 2000; Des Jarlais, 1995; International harm reduction association – IHRA, https://hri.global/?no-splash=true, now called Harm reduction international). The UK was notable for its harm reduction centres (e.g. Merseyside), in a context of increasing intravenous drug use. This strategy was adopted in diverse contexts, including needle exchange and methadone programs seen as effective strategies to reduce infectious disease transmission and decrease related mortality (Wodak, 1995; Merson et al., 2000; Gibson et al., 2001; Mattick et al., 2003a, 2003b *apud* Hunt & Stevens, 2004, p. 335).

Another important debate regards harm reduction related to psychiatric drugs. Self-organised groups of patients and survivors of psychiatric treatment (as some self-identity), together with professionals, have organised meetings, conferences and publications providing information about psychiatric drugs, how to get off them, and indications for best practice clinics and self-help groups. A series of networks were organised challenging mainstream psychiatric views and providing support in the UK, such as Survivors Speak Out, and in 1990s the National Self-Harm Network (feminist influence), Mad Pride, the Hearing Voices (Gordo-López, 2002) and the Paranoia Network (Parker, 2007). I highlight in England *Asylum: The Magazine for Democratic Psychiatry*[8] has campaigned against psychiatrisation and stigmatisation since 1986 and has been offering information and providing space for the users' perspective.[9]

Several studies (Stimson, 2000; Hunt & Stevens, 2004) highlight numerous measures during the late 1990s and early 2000s that shifted drug policy perspectives from health to crime. Drugs were seen as an 'engine of crime' (Hunt & Stevens, 2004, p. 334), while maintaining drug prevention as strategy in the UK and elsewhere. Before attention was given to drug use and HIV infection, the risk of self-harm and a risk to society by increasing disease was the focus. The focus then moved to criminality and harm to others (Hunt & Stevens, 2004), which is the main approach today. McSweeney et al. (2006) argue that these measures impose greater restrictions on low-risk offenders, and enforcement of penalties is contributing to a growing prison population.

This shift is seen in the new measures for compulsory and quasi-compulsory drug treatment that have been implemented in the UK and USA and in other countries (Netherlands, Germany, Brazil, among others). Drug Courts were first developed in the USA and partially informed the development of DTTOs (drug treatment and testing orders) (Hunt & Stevens, 2004). Concern was raised (McSweeney et al., 2006; Hunt & Stevens, 2004) over compulsory and quasi-compulsory treatment, in terms of ethics, human rights and effectiveness. In Brazil, compulsory or quasi-compulsory treatment was implemented, with many of these treatment centres having an Evangelical (47%) and/or Catholic (27%) religious foundation (IPEA, 2017 *apud* Targino, 2021), while obstacles to implement harm reduction policies have been documented (Figueiredo & Cavallari, 2020). Studies have also highlighted this shift in other countries, such as Russia (Margo, 2016).

It is crucial for public policy and research to account for social and individual contexts, considering gender, class, race, age, sexuality, disability, drug type and mode of consumption. For example, there is a notable lack of research on the use of solvents as drugs in Brazil, a gap in the literature that could be resolved with adequate attention to these criteria (Mountian, 2013a). Moreover, the use of psychiatric drugs, such as anti-depressants, is an important area of research. The 2010 United Nations Commission on

Narcotic Drugs expressed concern over the use of prescription drugs as seen in the increase in psychotropic drug consumption. Studies have highlighted international trends of higher prescription of psychotropic drugs for women and the elderly, and those from lower socio-economic groups (Cooperstock & Parnell, 2002; Ettorre & Riska, 1995; Lopes, 1999). Moore et al. (2009) highlight the increase of anti-depressant prescriptions in England, Australia and Canada, where women were more diagnosed with depression than men and showing an increase among young women between 1993 and 2005. Furthermore, previous research has observed an over prescription of anti-depressants for some groups of asylum seekers in the UK (Dawson, 2003) and the need to research these prescriptions for female asylum seekers (Mountian, 2005).

The effects of the prohibition of specific drugs have effects into the way that drugs are conceived and used. According to several studies, despite punishment and law enforcement, the consumption (in the UK, Birdwell et al., 2011) and production of illegal drugs (McSweeney et al., 2008) increased, while a large number of new drugs have been created (Birdwell et al., 2011). Studies highlight the effects of prohibition (Karam, 2008), such as violence, repression, misinformation, lack of drug quality control and health hazards for users (information, drug quality, risk of infection from diseases such as HIV and hepatitis), and how the effects of this legislation can be more harmful to the individual than the drugs themselves (Inciardi & Harrison, 2000). Reports also emphasise the need for more research into the new drugs and how technology and global markets are changing patterns of drug use (Reuter, 2011, also check UN report, 2024). It is important to consider local cultures and specificities given the implementation of a universal law (Rodrigues, 2003). Facing these challenges, drug policy is currently being reviewed, and new legislation has been enacted to relax laws, particularly for marihuana, as seen in Uruguay, USA, Canada and others.

Deconstructing drug addiction

Here I focus on a critical analysis of the notion of addiction, a fundamental term in the field of drug policy. For this, it is important to note that while I do not deny the experience of addiction or mental suffering and also seek to analyse how discourses on drug addiction are used, aiming to consider other discursive alternatives. As Loose (2002b, p. 273) emphasises, drawing on the work of Zafiropoulos, 'addiction exists, but there is no such person as *the* (typical) addict'. It is crucial to consider the social context and the relation of the subject to the substance, given that focusing solely on chemical effects prevents a broader understanding of drug use.

Defining addiction is crucial for public policy on prevention and treatment; however, these are often ambiguous or contradictory, in fact, 'the history of addiction came to be equated to the history of drug control' (Zieger, 2008). As Bucher (1992) points out regarding drug addiction (*toxicomania*) everything is problematic, starting with the word itself.[10] Addiction has become a term used to diagnose many types of behaviour in popular and medical language. Szasz (1975) reminds us that 'addiction' meant a strong inclination towards certain kinds of behaviour with little or no pejorative meaning attached to it. Among pre-20th-century examples found in the Oxford English Dictionary, Szasz (1975) observed addictions to civil affairs, to useful reading, as well as to bad habits. Nowadays, it refers 'to almost any kind of illegal, immoral, or undesirable association with certain kinds of drugs' (Szasz, 1975, p. 6).

The notion of addiction started to be developed by the end of the 19th century and beginning of the 20th. From 1897, articles began to utilise the terms such as 'drug habit', 'drug addiction' and 'drug patients' (mainly in North American and British journals) (Parascandola, 1996), after the First World War the association between drugs and abuse became widespread.

Medical discourses surrounding addiction have become popularised, indicating behaviours seen as 'excessive, habitually repetitive, or problematic' (White, 2004, p. 42), referring to compulsive behaviour towards specific 'objects' and activities (e.g. psychoactive substances, food, gym, televisions, computer, games and even sex and people). These include sex addiction, workaholism, shopaholics, chocoholics, caffeine addiction, eating addiction and gym addiction. Sedgwick (1992, p. 584) comments on practices regarded as addictive such as 'workaholism', 'shopaholism', 'sexual compulsiveness', 'co-dependency' or 'relationship addiction', such that 'as each assertion of will has made volition itself appear problematic in a new area, the assertion of will itself has come to appear addictive'.

The World Health Organisation (WHO) defines addiction as:

> Addiction refers to the repeated use of a psychoactive substance or substances, to the extent that the user is *periodically* or chronically intoxicated, shows a compulsion to take the preferred substance (or substances), has great difficulty in voluntarily ceasing or modifying substance use, and *exhibits determination to obtain psychoactive substances by almost any means.*
>
> (Lexicon of Alcohol and Drug Terms, WHO, 1994, p. 10, p. 73, my emphasis)

This definition does not specify the levels of 'determination' required, the types of substances and what form of use is included in this definition. However, this definition came to imply illegal or very expensive ones (Szasz, 1994). This definition appears as contrasting to 'habituation', that is, to become accustomed to any behaviour or condition, which discursively implies a socially accepted use of drugs (Young, 1971). In fact, the notion of habit can be seen to lose its place in drug debates, as Sedgwick (1992, p. 591) notes 'the worldly concept of habit has dropped out of theorised use with the superinvention in this [20th] century of addiction and the other glamorising paradigms oriented around absolutes of compulsion/volition'.

The Diagnostic and Statistical Manual of Mental Disorders (DSM), published by the American Psychiatric Association (APA), and the Classification of Mental and Behavioural Disorders (ICD 10), published by World Health Organisation (WHO), define drug dependence in relation to physical and psychological dependence, understanding it as a mental illness. Dependency is another term utilised for the definition of addiction,[11] yet this conceptualisation remains vague, and crucially, individual differences and social contexts are not ignored, discursively implying a difference between medical and recreational use. Dependency is typically seen as an undesirable aspect of human behaviour, conceived as less natural, less 'healthy' or less satisfying, commonly regarded as an undesirable quality, and in some discourses as a form of 'bondage' or 'slavery', as previously highlighted. Drawing on Dean and Taylor-Gooby's (1992) discussion of the underclass and welfare dependency, the meanings evoked by 'dependency' can be seen to connote a lack of power. The term is also highly gendered, with autonomy regarded as the cultural ideal of Western masculinity and dependence as attributed to the feminised 'Other'. Addiction and dependency are notions that must be located in their specific social and historical contexts.

The moral connotation of drug dependency is further reviewed, as pointed out by McDonald (1994, p. 3): 'it is still the case that the imputed "addictiveness" of a substance holds a persuasive congruence with the degree of religious and political fear of it, and the capacity for evil attributed to it'. Katz (1997) debates how secular values of health came to replace non-corporeal or theological virtues, constituting a 'new morality', operating discursively by supplementing the traditional moral code related to sin and redemption. Health came to be related to the way people behave implying notions such as moral character and self-control.

In this sense, a deconstruction of the word 'chemical' highlights its negative connotation, contrasting with discourses of the body as organic and natural (Keane, 1999), or pure. Here, it is interesting to note the notions of natural and artificial as described by Irigaray (1989 *apud* Frosh, 1995), wherein natural is seen as cyclical and organic, while artificial is labyrinthine, being therefore subjected to law, as is the case with drugs.

Other debates highlight the discursive implications of the notion of dependency and the production of specific polarised aspects. The notion of dependency appears in contrast to free-will (Davies, 1997), such that specific choices are discursively understood as a non-choice. This definition of addiction 'resides only in the structure of a will that is always somehow insufficiently free, a choice whose volition is insufficiently pure' (Sedgwick, 1992, p. 584). This lack provides the material for the definition of addiction, as Sedgwick (1992) argues, 'the object of addiction is the exercise of those very qualities whose lack is supposed to define addiction as such: bodily autonomy, self-control, will power'. It is worth considering Keane's (1999) insights inspired in Derrida, which emphasise how the attachment to pleasure is held against the drug user. The objection is not about the pleasure of the user *per se*, but 'we cannot abide that this is a pleasure taken in an experience without truth' (Keane, 1999, p. 70).

Legitimacy becomes related to the opposition between natural and artificial (Carneiro, 2019), true and false, pure and impure, legitimate and illegitimate pleasures, and legitimate free will. This perspective on addiction provides a discursive division between false and real pleasures, 'in which the inauthenticity of the drug addict is chemically produced and objectively verifiable' (Mountian, 2013a). Sedgwick (1992, p. 589) drawing on The Picture of Dorian Gray and Dr. Jekyll and Mr. Hyde (erotic tension between men and solitary substance abusers) highlights how:

> The two new taxonomies of the addict and the homosexual condensed many of the same issues for late nineteenth-century culture: the old-anti-sodomitic opposition between something called 'nature' and that which is *contra naturam* blended with a treacherous apparent seamlessness into a new opposition between substances that are natural (for example, 'food') and those that are artificial (for example, 'drugs'), and hence into the characteristic twentieth century way of distinguishing desires themselves between the natural, called 'need', and the artificial, called 'addictions'.

Queer theories further the debate on the legitimacy of body and pleasure, and on the relation of ethics to pleasure and the definition of freedom (Warner, 1999). An understanding of homosexuality as well as drug use as medical conditions provided the medical perspective with a specific discursive space for legitimacy.

The impact of the mental health classification of addiction and how drug policies came to operate will be further analysed in Chapter 5, focusing on the social imaginary of women and drugs and pointing out how gender, race, sexuality and age are viewed within drug discourses.

Final remarks

This chapter focused on the history of the psychiatric diagnosis of depression, hysteria, homosexuality, transsexuality and drug addiction. A socio-historical perspective on the definition of mental disorders also reveals the therapeutic culture that is produced. Some aspects are important to be highlighted here: first an awareness of hasty associations between mental disorders and minoritised groups, as seen in the case of depression and other mental disorders, in relation to women, black people and migrants; second, how situated cultural and moral values interpolate the production of mental health classifications regarding specific groups, such as the history of homosexualism and transsexualism as mental illness; and third, how moral values are imbedded in the mental health classifications, the consequent production of legislation according to medical discourses and the effects on minoritised groups, as in the case of drugs, as seen from treatment to legislation, which has specific effects on women, LGBTQI+ people, black people, working class and impoverished people and migrants.

Notes

1 Translation by the author
2 Translated by the author
3 https://www.euro.who.int/en/health-topics/health-determinants/gender/gender-definitions/whoeurope-brief-transgender-health-in-the-context-of-icd-11#:~:text=ICD%2D11%20has%20redefined%20gender,incongruence%20of%20childhood%E2%80%9D%2C%20respectively
4 Translation by the author, from informal media
5 The word narcotic comes from the Greek *narkoun* meaning to sleep or sedate (Escohotado, 1998). Although the World Health Organisation classifies narcotic drugs in medicine as a 'chemical agent that induces stupor, coma, or insensibility to pain (also called narcotic analgesic)' (United Nations Office for Drug Control and Drug Prevention, 2003, Internet), in contemporary discourses, this term is applied for a wide range of drugs.
6 The 1972 UN Convention amended that of 1961 to include drugs not present in the latter. The classification became: list 1 – hallucinogenic drugs, list 2 – amphetamines, list 3 and 4 – different types of barbiturates. Only the drugs from list 1 were completely prohibited for supposedly possessing no medical function.
7 It is relevant to highlight the context of the emergence of AIDS and the impact on drug policy, having more campaigns targeting LGBTQI+ people and women (also including in prostitution), often seen as possible transmitters. Studies (Prado & Machado, 2008) point out the stigmatisation of homosexual people with the association with HIV and drug use.
8 See www.asylumonline.net
9 See discourseunit.com
10 Translated by the author
11 'Drug dependence' in the UN definition means: 'a cluster of physiological, behavioural and cognitive phenomena of variable intensity, in which the use of a psychoactive drug (or drugs) takes on a high priority. It implies a need for repeated doses of the drug to feel good or avoid feeling bad'. 'Psychological or psychic dependence' refers to the experience of impaired control over drug use. 'Physiological or physical dependence' involves the development of tolerance and withdrawal symptoms upon cessation of use of the drug, as a consequence of the body's adaptation to the continued presence of a drug (Laboratory and Scientific Section United Nations Office on Drugs and Crime, 2003, p. 74).

Part II

To practice

Researching mental health

In this second part of the book, I concentrate on debates resulting from the research I conducted in Brazil and England. The aspects covered in the first part provide the epistemological background and primary insights for our analysis of the relationship between mental health and otherness, particularly for the inclusion of the social context and the position of the Other as subject in psy practice and theory. These are relevant when analysing how minoritised groups are (mis)interpreted and (mis)represented in research and practice. On one hand, the effects of an objectified view of the Other are observed in practice, while on the other, through encounters it may be possible to contextualise psy-disciplines and to deconstruct the fetishised view of the Other, allowing for a possible broader understanding of health and mental health.

In the following chapters, I will present some of this research, focusing on the intersections between gender, race, sexuality, age, and class and how these operate in the field of mental health. As seen in the first part of the book, a critical reflexivity towards research practice is fundamental, with aspects of reflexivity and the positionality of the researcher being approached in different ways. Although in this publication I will not be able to extend this analysis, I will indicate some of these issues in my research, during which most of the fieldwork was carried out in partnership with the groups directly involved in the study, such as interviews conducted by *travestis*, by health service providers, workshops led by immigrants, meetings with immigrant organisations and analysis of the position of the psychologist in the research with drug users.

In Chapter 3 I will focus on the research into immigration and mental health, highlighting issues involving the encounter between immigrants, including young people, and health service providers in the UK and Brazil. This raises questions regarding the discursive position of the immigrant, as a symbolic position of the Other, and the situated understanding of health and mental health.

Chapter 4 will focus on issues related to older *travestis*, and transgender and transsexual women in Brazil. The way intersectional categories operate

DOI: 10.4324/9780429263415-5

in this context is highlighted, showing how transphobia operates, thereby hindering possibilities for social inclusion and access to health services. Further, the dynamics of (in)visibility of older and younger trans people (and non-binary people) in health and mental health services and in public spaces more generally raise important concerns to be considered in psy-disciplines.

Returning to the issues previously considered in Chapter 2, Chapter 5 will focus on the intersections between gender, sexuality, age, class and drug use. The way women are viewed in the field of drugs reproduces the social position of women, while drug policy and treatment centres are conceived of through a masculine lens having the male the main subject for intervention. The dynamics of visibility and invisibility of women and LGBTQIA+ people and drug use will be further analysed, highlighting the importance of socially inclusive drug policy.

In the final chapter 'conclusions', I will discuss how these studies put into question the situatedness of our conceptions of health and mental health in psy-disciplines, showing how these frequently reproduce determined understandings of the Other, within processes of minoritising given communities. Both in practice and theory, and within a critical perspective, it therefore becomes crucial to interrogate how we listen to the Other. This can be seen in the process whereby through the encounter, where the Other is conceived, both the Us and the Them are produced. From this perspective, I review the possibilities of interrogating and transforming the fetishised position of the Other, seeking a listening that permits the emergence of the subject (both of desire and knowledge).

3 Immigration, gender and mental health in England and Brazil

This chapter will present insights arising from the research projects on immigration and health and mental health that I undertook in the UK and Brazil from 2005 to 2018. The analysis shows how understandings of mental health are culturally located revealing a situated therapeutic culture, and how it is crucial to consider the social context of immigration during clinical work. Three main aspects are highlighted: first, the importance of considering how social constraints affect mental health; second, how minoritised communities access health services; and third, how conceptions of gender and race in the immigration context impact the practice and theory of mental health and health.

From the fieldwork conducted, we firstly emphasise the risks of resorting to hasty psychiatric diagnoses of immigrants, without considering the social conditions they experience, which can produce a number of consequences for the subject, from stigmatisation to the effects of prescribed psychiatric drugs. The psychiatrisation of immigrants (and women) can discursively produce a naturalisation of mental health issues, "naturalising" the subject's condition as a bio-physiological given, rather than understanding it within the relevant social relations, in this case, overlooking the processes of immigration themselves. Regarding the second aspect, it is important to analyse the accessibility of services to immigrants, from cultural sensitivity to possibilities of access to health services (including information). Thirdly, it is crucial to recognise how conceptions of gender and race in the immigration context affect the practice and theory of mental health and health, situating the conceptions of 'women' and LGBTQIA+ people within health services, the social position of the 'migrant women' and 'migrant LGBTQIA+ people', consequent forms of settling and impact into health and mental health.

It becomes clear that the concept of health and mental health are not neutral or universal, that is, different understandings of the body are at play in different cultures (not only related to foreign countries), which directly affects the treatment of immigrants. It is important to consider the effects of these views on women, extending the analysis to LGBTQIA+ people, within the specific constraints according to the social context. This analysis requires an intersectional perspective encompassing gender, sexuality, race, class, age and

DOI: 10.4324/9780429263415-6

disability, for the encounter between health services and minoritised groups (Chantler et al., 2003; Chantler, 1998); otherwise, it risks reproducing stereotypical views on minoritised groups. Fernando (2012) points out that services were criticised for not respecting and being out of touch with the Black and Ethnic Minority communities, seen particularly in the notion of mental health that overlooks cultural diversity. Dialogue with the service-user is inadequately integrated and valued, with little participation from the user. Moreover, the importance of service provisions for migrant women, especially victims of domestic violence, is highlighted here.

In the following sections, I will further explore these aspects through the research undertaken with asylum seekers and refugees in England and Brazil, including: *Young asylum seekers, refugees and drug use* (Early Break, Manchester Metropolitan University, Rochdale Homelessness, Home Office), *Women Asylum Seekers from Pakistan who seek refugee protection in the UK against domestic violence* (Manchester Metropolitan University) and *Asylum seekers and refugees' access to health service in Manchester* (Manchester Primary Care Trust, Manchester Metropolitan University). In Brazil, the research projects were: *Otherness and migration: intersecting gender, race and class* (Universidade de São Paulo, FAPESP grants), and *Intersectionality and Otherness: trajectories of immigration and social networks* (Casa do Migrante and OPAS/WHO, Universidade de Sao Paulo, Capes/PNPD grants). During the period of this latter study, I had the opportunity to coordinate a project tackling xenophobia, racism and sexism in the Sao Paulo public health system, commissioned by the Sao Paulo Town Hall and OPAS/WHO, which I will draw upon here. Moreover, the analysis also reflects my participation in the health network for immigrants in Sao Paulo since 2012 and the supervision for the clinical intervention at the Casa do Migrante (Scalabrinian temporary shelter for immigrants in Sao Paulo[1]). I provide an overview of the research projects in Appendix 1.

3.1 Immigration processes and mental health in the UK

This section focuses on the importance for health and mental health theory and practice of considering the immigrant's social context. For this, health and mental health practice and theory, particularly when working with minoritised groups, require constant critical reflexivity. In the research conducted on immigrants and health services, we observed the need to consider the social context and the intersectional dynamics of key social categories of gender, sexuality, race, age, class and disability, to comprehend discourses surrounding asylum seekers and refugees. How these aspects are considered is at stake in the analysis of health and mental health practice. When we understand mental health problems as an isolated issue of an individual immigrant abstracted from the broader context within which they live, the diverse factors that generate stressful conditions and requiring interrogation become normalised. While the individual's mental health struggles and suffering must be considered, their social context also needs to be fully recognised, given that the context has a direct effect on the subject and ultimately for the medical diagnosis.

Immigration processes are heterogeneous, presenting diverse challenges, uncertainties, unforeseen difficulties and possibilities for change. This process has to be situated according to the social power relations, and economic, political and cultural specificities, which impact the subject in multiple ways. Diasporas have complex histories, compounded by different and multiple journeys, specificities and narratives (Brah, 1996). As Brah (1996, p. 180) argues, 'the concept of diaspora centres on the *configurations of power which differentiate diasporas internally as well as situate them in relation to one another*'.

Diasporas are heterogeneous and a critical eye towards attempts to homogenise individual experience is necessary. In the same vein, it becomes important to consider the discursive processes through which the collective 'we' is produced (Brah, 1996). Processes of immigration must be understood by considering differences of class, gender, age, race, sexuality and disability that will play a major role in the diverse forms of immigration and settlement. The feminisation of immigration (and of poverty) brings a number of issues to account for (care, social mobility, family structure), as well as differences in immigration for women, children and adolescents (Duarte et al., 2019).

The form of settlement necessitates an analysis of encounters between the immigrant and the hosting society, which will determine a range of possibilities for the subject, considering how specific forms of violence might also occur, such as xenophobia, racism, sexism and classism. In this sense, the first aspect to interrogate regards the specific social dynamics in which the subject is embedded, and how distributions of power operate, including within the field of health.

The process of displacement and settlement is not the same for each individual, and there are great differences according to the countries' immigration controls and forms of processing and reception. As Brah (1996) suggests, 'the identity of the diasporic imagined community is far from fixed or pre-given. It is constituted within the crucible of the materiality of everyday life; in the everyday stories we tell ourselves individually and collectively'. In accordance with the malleability of culture, rather than focusing on the fixed identity of the immigrant, attention is given to the social conditions, and on how the signifier 'culture' operates for both the subject and service providers. The concern here is with immigration processes that are often filled with uncertainties, growing bureaucratic hardships, and separation from family members and basic social networks, particularly for asylum seekers and refugees.

In previous research (Mountian, 2005, 2015, 2020; Fang et al., 2015), some issues associated with the experience of asylum seekers and refugees were identified, such as obstacles to accessing basic rights (housing, health, work and education), different reasons and forms of migration (forced migration, war, political upheaval, persecution and torture), challenges of settlement (changes in legislation), violence (racism, sexism, social exclusion), isolation and stigmatisation (Patel, 2004). As Harradine (2004) emphasises, these aspects, which can increase an individual's vulnerability, require a local community response for asylum seekers, accounting for the specifics of the situation, in order to avoid leaving them impoverished and isolated. Regarding drug use, previous reports (Dawson, 2003; The Mayor of London, 2004) highlight that depending on the culture of the country of origin, asylum seekers may never have used drugs prior to their arrival (Dawson, 2003), which was also seen in the research on young people (Mountian, 2005), although there was a concern regarding over-prescription of tranquilisers for women (often their mothers).

Within this context, it is relevant to highlight the difficulties and complexities surrounding research on sensitive themes such as immigration, drug use and others. In these research settings, the way that secrecy and silence operate has to be analysed, from the avoidance of talking about difficult issues to the sensitivity in researching groups that face authority decisions (Mountian, 2005).

This contextualisation brings challenges to service providers, as seen when 'there is a need to explore the broader determinants of health. . . . Emphasis must be placed on addressing associated macro-level structural factors' (Fang et al., 2015, p. 16). From this, some aspects can already be underlined as important for service provision: a) awareness of services immigrants can access, b) fear of deportation may play an important role when disclosing confidential issues, c) language barriers and d) effects of past and present traumatic experiences, including racial and gendered dynamics.

Deconstructing discourses on immigration

Immigration is not a new event in history; however, immigration control and registration are contemporary, enacted during the 20th century. In the UK, the 1905 Aliens Act was the first immigration control act, associated with Jewish people fleeing Polish and Russian pogroms. This was followed by the 1962 Commonwealth Immigration Act, the 1971 Immigration Act, the 1981 British Nationality Act and the 2002 Nationality, Immigration and Asylum Act referring to people seeking asylum, among others.

Cohen (2001) highlights how immigration control intersects with race and class distinctions, seen for example in the 1905 Aliens Act, applied to the poorest immigrants, to those on the first- or second-class travel facilities. In this context, discourses on the social cost of Jewish refugees started to emerge, which in fact has some resonance with current discourses on asylum seekers. Support was given to those who could improve the British economy and were unlikely to use welfare. For application rulings, focus was given to undesirability, more precisely to 'the diseased, the insane, the criminal and those likely to be a burden on the public purse'. However, 'medical rejections were often quite vague, reflecting a concern with economic productivity without recourse to the public purse' (Hayes, 2004, p. 18). Likewise, by 1882 the US had banned immigration by mentally ill people, which meant people who could develop symptoms within one year of arrival, and later within three years, if they could demonstrate that these symptoms were related to conditions prior to the immigration (Littlewood & Lipsedge, 2001). In the 20th century, this ban extended to alcoholics, psychopaths and illiterate people (2001).

In the 1990s, the category 'asylum seeker' was specified in UK legislation, in the 1993 Asylum Immigration Appeals Act; the 1996 Asylum, Immigration Act and the 1999 Immigration and Asylum Act. Wren (2007) argues that the 1999 Immigration Asylum Act instituted a key change in the way asylum seekers were supported in the UK. This act 'separates the social rights of asylum seekers from those of other UK citizens and non-citizen residents (primarily to deter economic migration)' (Wren, 2007, p. 393). 'Welfare rights may vary considerably depending on date of entry; those lodging "in-country claims" more than 72 hours after entry effectively have no right to public support; they are not allowed to work (since July 2002), no rights to family reunion' (Dwyer & Brown, 2005, p. 370).

Asylum seekers refer to people looking for protection in a new country, due to fear of persecution and make a claim for refugee status. According to the United Nations Convention on Refugees (1951), Article 1A a refugee is a person

> who has a well-founded fear of persecution due to race, religion, nationality, political opinion or membership of a particular social group or political opinion, is outside the country of his nationality and is unable or, owing to such fear, is unwilling to avail himself of the protection of that country; or who, not having a nationality and being outside the country of his former habitual residence as a result of such events, is unable or, owing to such fear, is unwilling to return to it.
>
> (UNHCR, 1996, p. 16 *apud* Patel, 2004, p. 16)

Refugee status guarantees the right to stay (work and access to basic rights) and to apply for settlement, then acquiring the same rights as national citizens.

Critical immigration studies argue that citizenship, defined by borders, keeps asylum seekers out of place. McMaster (2003) observes that they are in the '"shadowlands" where the abstract construct of citizenship is changing but the legal-political constructs are not' (p.1), they do "not belong", but rather are positioned at the margins. As Spybey emphasises: 'the nation-state and the nation-state system have rendered citizenship a universal requirement for the legal sanction of human existence; a stateless person does not exist in legal terms' (Spybey, 1996, p. 169). However, stateless persons do exist, and their numbers are rising due to global events. 'Citizenship as a legal national identity requirement has become a universal, but this does not construct universal citizenship nor provide human rights' (McMaster, 2003, p. 7).

It is important to analyse how discourses on race operate within processes of immigration, settlement and citizenship. Hayes (2004) claims that specific groups of people are racialised and presented as a threat to the receiving nation, in terms of material resources and culture, maintaining them as 'outsiders'. This construction of the racialised Other is socially situated, as race (and gender) is produced over time, it has a history that is reproduced through discourse. It becomes important to analyse the performativity of race, given by the repetition of acts and its stickiness, consolidating in specific discourses. As Butler (1997, p. 140) suggests, 'one speaks a language that is never fully one's own, but that language only persists through repeated occasions of that invocation'.

Discourses on asylum seekers were seen to (re)produce specific stereotypes, often with negative connotations, for example 'bogus', 'beggars', 'arrest' (Tait, 2004), having overtaken the humanitarian imperative of providing asylum, frequently seen as a liability rather than as an asset for society (The Mayor of London, 2004, p. 57). Discourses around asylum seekers often bring up issues surrounding racism and poverty, categories that must be considered in their intersection, and understanding the asylum process itself as, in some cases, leading to impoverishment. It is relevant to analyse how the signifiers' asylum seeker and refugee appear and are used in discourse, placing asylum seekers in specific positions, and how these affect treatment and health services. The social imaginary position occupied by immigrants can often be seen in the polarised discourses of the 'victim' and the 'threat', thereby reifying the subject. What other possible discursive positions can asylum seekers occupy?

Moreover, it is worthwhile to reflect on the social functions of fear. Ahmed (2003) suggests that fear is not conceived simply as an individual matter, but rather has a social role, aligning individuals with communities. The role of emotions is 'sticking figures together (adherence), a stickiness that creates the very effect of a collective (coherence)' (2003, p. 2). Emotions are economic; 'they circulate between signifiers in relationships of difference and displacement' (2003). By naming the fear (see also Badiou, 2001), there is a fantasy of managing the enemy of it, being easier to bear it. As psychoanalysis reveals 'by naming what is going on, we cease to be ravished by it' (Frosh, 1995, p. 296). Here it is posed the question on the discursive space of 'asylum seekers'.

Becoming asylum seeker: contextualising young people and family

I will present some emergent issues from the study of young people and drug use (Mountian, 2005), such as the hardship of the asylum-seeking processes, language, the role of family and life circumstances. Aiming to outline some of these aspects, I will present extracts from the interviews with service providers. In the following interview, a broader view of the social context of young asylum seekers and refugees is highlighted:

> By their nature and because of what they have gone through it is not very easy at first to [form relationship] because they have been through a lot

and they may have been told not to talk about things. . . . Once they know people in our dept things do come out. Because they come in the room and they sit and they chat and things come out. You do find out things, it is a long time before they will trust an adult because in some way they have been abused in the (pause). . . . Erm and they . . . are a little bit insecure even the ones from the most secure backgrounds because they have been uprooted and planted somewhere else and erm the asylum process does not help (big sigh), that they don't know if they are going to stay here, they know that their parents are worried, they know that their parents are seeing solicitors and sometimes they have to go down to London to see solicitors and they are backward and forward which adds to their sense of insecurity. . . . Until they get their leave to stay here. . . . Which very few people get, they are up in the air about their positions and it is difficult to console them cos you can't give them any reassurances, we don't know if they will have to go back (6)

A lot of children have to do the translating for their parents so they know all about it. . . . We have had children who have become mentally ill because of the stresses they are going through. . . . It's upsetting for me never mind them, to see a child break down is awful. . . . A lot of them are the carers of their parents, some of the parents may not have told them what they have gone through in their own country, but the kids realise that their parents are not the parents that they started off with shall we say. . . . Some of the parents suffer some sort of mental illness and some of the kids become the carers, partly because their English is better, but sometimes just having to be more responsible, looking after the shopping, looking after younger siblings, sorting out appointments, making phone calls, asking relevant questions and a lot of them are, . . . have very old heads on their shoulders because of what has happened in the past. . . . Which is . . . Sad. That's the nature of them. (6)

In this extract, the hardships of 'becoming an asylum seeker' are highlighted, including isolation, fear and insecurity. As such, past experiences and the present asylum-seeking process must be considered for young people and their family. In this extract, the difficulties faced by the family, which occupy a central role for young people, show the impact on the individual's mental health. The social context in which the young people, family and carers act alongside immigration and settlement processes must be considered, as further pressure might be present. Issues regarding the role of interpreters were also highlighted, demanding an adult attitude from the young people for translation, an aspect that will be further discussed later on.

A lot of the time with adults you are meeting them in a new environment and there is a lot of anxiety and concerns that the parents have got about the safety of professionals especially if you are in a situation where the family are feeling they are under threat of being arrested and

> being deported. Erm . . . so . . . generally I think children are quite isolated anyway isolated and don't have much contact and I think most of them respond well to offers if it is appropriate to them but I guess they have to want to see somebody.
>
> (7)
>
> F. – Right. . . . Do you think that is to do with the background they have come from?
>
> I think well perhaps less of the background and more to do with the current situation where they are under . . . under . . . where they have to behave trying to get their status worked out so it's a compulsion to follow the rules.
>
> (7)

Here, we see the effect of the asylum seeker's context at work, where fear of deportation, uncertainty about the refugee process and the future of their family are at stake. These aspects are important to be taken into account in the relationship with the young people and professionals, as fear of authority can play a part in the confidence in professionals (Franks et al., 2007). The following extract highlights some aspects of family dynamics in this context.

An example of a knock on effect is you might have older siblings who might have to care for the younger siblings because their parents are incapable getting up a lot of the time and doing things, so you find that an older sibling is getting up in the morning and taking the younger ones to school and they take on a paternal role, sometimes we will go round to see a family and we will find them, in the middle of the day in bed, very very tired with the curtains drawn and yet they are not sleeping they are just kind of existing in that depressed state really and then obviously the children, they don't get the interaction or a lot of the things children need to flourish so.

(5)

Here the impact of the asylum-seeking process on the adult's mental health and on the children's familial role is highlighted.

> My impressions are that they are very vulnerable in a lot of ways, although they learn English a lot quicker than their parents and pick up the language quicker, it's the people that they meet in schools, some of our children get involved with the wrong kind of young people in school, some of them are getting themselves into trouble. Part of that is that some of our young people have behaviour problems because of issues cos of stuff that has happened to them in the past back home, because of the conflict. It's just like minor things, but I see them as being really vulnerable because they don't really have a clue what society is like here, especially the girls. The girls are much protected.
>
> (1)

The vulnerability of young people was highlighted during this research. While young people showed greater ease of language acquisition, adaptation to new environments was seen as a challenge, alongside the effects of past experiences. Issues around bullying are crucial to address, and the need to specify the type of bullying experienced by young people (e.g. racist bullying). Further, there is a need to investigate if reporting bullying to the police is seen as a safe strategy for asylum seekers. Cultural differences related to gender was emphasised in the following extract:

> I feel that the amount of power somebody can have to damage somebody's reputation can be quite harrowing, especially within a community that has a culture of bringing young women up as, I don't think I mean subservient, but bring young women up to be in the home, to look after the home, to help Mum do whatever, until she is found a husband so she can be married, but when you get the impact of er words and people feeling that they have been wronged and how you can damage somebody's reputation with that is quite worrying.
>
> (8)

Concern about young women is expressed in this extract, raising important issues for consideration. It is relevant to analyse how discourses on gender and culture operate within the immigration process. While the social dynamics of patriarchal cultures must be acknowledged and tackled, the way that gender and culture overlap must be carefully interrogated, as at times, it can invoke a fixed and stereotypical idea of culture, while it might discursively position *their* culture, through gender, in a devalued place, contrasting to *our* culture (McClintock, 1995), leaving gender violence within non-western cultures unchallenged (Soans, 2015). These juxtapositions of gender and culture operate in diverse ways, creating challenges for service providers.

Moreover, cultural differences with Western cultures are also expressed through the parent-child generation gap. The intersection between culture and age is important, as new adaptations are required from the family and service providers.

Language, culture and service provision: elements for service provision

Culture is an important aspect to be taken into account when developing services; in some instances, 'culture' was mentioned as a barrier to access asylum seekers. However, what culture is and how it is constituted must be critically analysed and considered in relation to the local culture, as the encounter also sheds light on 'our' own culture. Culture is commonly used with a specific meaning or encompassing people from a specific geographic area. A broader perspective is needed, as people from the same locality might have little in common (e.g. social and political backgrounds, race, class, gender, religion). Services also need to ensure not taking for granted, naturalising or normalising exceptional circumstances (e.g. war, asylum seeking process) as part of a culture.

The importance of being culturally sensitive was emphasised, and a multi-racial task force was indicated by service providers as the best approach to services, as the same culture service provider may create other sorts of issues, such as reproducing specific power imbalances. For the implementation of these strategies, some considerations were highlighted regarding issues surrounding confidentiality, and opposing political orientation as these service providers may live in the same communities. However, in general, culturally specific services do make an important contribution within the overall framework of service development. As such, it was found that teams in the organisations should themselves be diverse groups, fully engaging with issues of race, class, gender and specifically immigration and asylum.

Language was mentioned as a barrier, as people may not speak the local language, and children were often acting as interpreters (e.g. at GP consultations), which raises another set of issues. An awareness about children as interpreters may be required, as there might be sensitive issues that parents and children did not previously expect to share. Regarding interpreters, some aspects were highlighted: The importance of providing translation of the information and having interpreters available for all circumstances related to access and delivery of services; the need to train interpreters for specific appointments (e.g. young people's health, child protection); an awareness of political differences between interpreters and clients; and the availability of clinical supervision for interpreters.

Some further suggestions arose from the research, such as the importance of services for 16 to 18 and 19 to 25 years old young asylum seekers, given that young adults may face different issues depending on age (e.g. education, deportation) and gender. Young people need to be aware they can access services, and the importance of counselling and psychological support, whether on the estates where they live, or through school. Furthermore, from the outcomes of this research, no specific need for a service for asylum seekers and refugees in terms of drug use was observed within the participant group; however, current services should be prepared to accommodate this population.[2]

From this research, it becomes clear the need for services to consider the intersections between age, gender, race, class and sexuality, considering the context of immigration. Initiatives from black and minority groups might be useful to think about services that encompass asylum seekers and refugees.

In this sense, the social context and dimensions related to the immigration process should be considered for mental health: first, in terms of the effect of such constraints on the subject and how mental health issues can be seen as a response for these challenging experiences, and second, how different understandings of mental health may impact treatment. These aspects will be further discussed next.

3.2 Asylum seekers' and refugees' access to health services and mental health issues

Considering the social context of asylum seekers and refugees, the process of immigration and adaptation to the host country emerge as conditions that can lead to further hardship for the subject. Here I will highlight some mental health and service provision dimensions that arose from the research *Asylum Seekers and Refugee's Access to Health Services* (2007). In the first part, I will focus on issues of distress and mental health among migrants, and in the second on challenges and approaches for health services.

As seen in previous research (Fang et al., 2015; Mountian, 2020), the discursive position of the immigrant as the Other reproduces a specific division between Us and Them, which overlaps with processes of marginalisation, stigmatisation and social exclusion. The way gender and sexuality operate through cultural ideals within these fields, which also affect processes of immigration and access to services, must be interrogated. The social imaginary surrounding asylum seekers and immigrants, characterising the intersectional categories of gender, sexuality, age and disability, was seen as having a significant impact on how health services engage with this population (Littlewood & Lipsedge, 1989; Hayes, 2004; The Mayor of London, 2004; Burman et al., 2004; Chantler et al., 2003).

Phoenix (1987) coined the term 'normalised absence, pathologised presence' for the exclusion of black people in research. Turning to the case of asylum seekers and refugees, it offers insights into the way dynamics of in/visibility operate in health services, particularly when their 'visibility becomes apparent only when their presence is problematized' (Fang et al., 2015, p. 15), that is, when seen as outside the norm, or as outsiders, deviant or pathological.

> [The] divide between 'us' and 'them,' which coincides with the concept of 'normalized absence, pathologized presence,' since the presence of the 'other' is often viewed as being intrusive whereas their absence is often preferred and widely accepted as being 'the norm' [9, 10]. Somali and Iraqi asylum seekers, refugees and individuals without legal status in the UK, are often stigmatized as being disingenuous, burdensome and a drain on resources [10] fitting the notion of 'pathologized presence.' Simultaneously, the process of 'normalized absence' often renders these individuals invisible in the health care system through the neglect of cultural and religious needs in health care policy.
>
> (Fang et al., 2015, pp. 15–16)

Interrogating the 'normalised absence and pathologised presence' of immigrants in health care provision, I will start by highlighting some mental health questions arising from the research conducted in Manchester on

Asylum Seeker and Refugee Access to health services (Fang et al., 2015). Many of the participants in the research spoke about mental health issues they had experienced or were then experiencing, with some reporting that they were suffering from depressive symptoms and expressing suicidal ideation. These symptoms were spoken associated with their past experiences and current social situation, which was understood as causing untold distress for asylum seekers and refugees. I will present some extracts of interviews with asylum seekers and refugees, in which they spoke about their struggles and experiences (e.g. war) before moving to the UK and present hardships.

> I think many of them, they are sad people. They have problems with their lives. They are irritable people and are mentally thinking all the time about their futures. Psychologically I think they are not good because they haven't any hopes with their lives, any sparkle, and they are afraid to send them back to Iraq for example. Always they are thinking about that and always thinking to send them back to Iraq because in Iraq their life was destroyed. They hadn't any food. They sold everything. They sold what they had, everything that they had possessed in their lives. If they go back to Iraq he thinks 'how can I do this again?' He has nothing. He sold his house, everything, he sold his shop, his business. Nothing. For that reason, obviously, he does not want to go back.[3]
>
> For me to be out of work affect me psychologically and I'm starting for the first time to experience depression and I'm afraid to stay for another one year, because now I can't return back penniless and I might be in danger also so I've seen some people like me, they've maybe been here two more years than me so I'm just afraid the longer to stay the more I will be depressed. The more I will delay to get indefinite [leave to remain] the more I will be depressed. I'm afraid of my health if I don't see my family soon.[4]
>
> I did not want to live because of what is gone. I was eating, sleeping only . . . I decided to forget it all, but it came back to my mind . . . I tried to forget it but I can't. My history, my life is stamped into my heart.[5]

In these extracts, the asylum-seeking process, impoverishment and the impossibility of work were aspects highlighted by the participants as stressful conditions, putting into question expectations for the future. The harmful impact of post-migratory issues on mental health has been documented, the asylum-seeking process, the fear of returning and refuse of asylum (BMA, 2002 *apud* Fell & Hayes, 2007; Morgan et al., 2017; Pollard & Howard, 2021). Moreover, research shows higher rates of mental illness among adult refugees, and long-term resettled refuges, anxiety and depression were related to poor social integration (Giacco & Priebe, 2018).

McColl and Johnson (2006) mapped mental health provision in London finding that 11% of Community Mental Health Team patients were asylum seekers or refugees. Co-morbidity was frequent, and psychiatrists reported significant diagnostic uncertainty for 30% of the diagnoses. The most common were depression (50%) and post-traumatic stress disorder (41%), with just over half presenting a psychotic diagnosis (53%). Social isolation was common, levels of unmet needs were high, and the group used few services other than the Community Mental Health Services. In Manchester based on the 2001 Census and the 1999 Health Survey for England, a higher incidence of psychiatric illness was also observed amongst South-Asian (Bangladesh, Pakistan, India) and Afro-Caribbean people.

This disproportional presence of minoritised groups underlines some important aspects to be further assessed. Firstly, how social conditions of asylum seekers and refugees impact mental health; secondly, the high rates of diagnostic uncertainty suggest a need for a clearer understanding of complex clinical syndromes alongside cultural attitudes and behaviours (Littlewood & Lipsedge, 2001); thirdly, attention should also be paid to over-prescription of anti-depressants to these groups, (Dawson, 2003) and lastly, a critical perspective regarding the diagnosis of immigrants is necessary, as stereotypes might be reproduced within the mental health field.

On one hand, it becomes paramount to socially contextualise the immigrant experience; while on the other, there are specificities that can be considered when working with asylum seekers and refugees. The assumption of health problems as individually situated without a broader social context implies the idea of an individual asylum seeker or refugee with their own individual problems to resolve, locating solutions at the individual level and assuming an individualised and Westernised construction of health. By separating the notion of reduced health inequality from individualised conceptions of health problems, one way forward may be, as Webster and Robertson (2007) argue, to focus more on the community level, providing services which are culturally congruent with the community's own health constructions. For this, the views of health service providers are as centrally important as those of asylum seekers and refugees themselves (Lau & Rodgers, 2021). The views of health service providers will be debated, in the case of Brazil, in sub-section 3.3.

On the second aspect, regarding the specificities and challenges of working with immigrants, there are issues from the immigrant experience that are important to consider, such as exceptional circumstances (war) and their effects (fear of persecution), the settlement process (uncertainties and constraints), the intersections of gender (women may be socially isolated and men may be isolated by language), race (xenophobia, discrimination and the effects of racism), religious practices (Littlewood & Lipsedge, 2001) and age and disability. Regarding gender, one also has to be aware of issues of gender abuse within familial contexts as well as traumatic events such as war rape. Research has consistently observed different culturally appropriate ways of defining and coping with explicit impairment (disability) and implicit impairment (mental health difficulties) (Roberts, 2000; Harris &Roberts, 2004; Webster & Robertson, 2007). These aspects have been taken on by

Black and Minority Ethnic (BME) agencies and research (Chantler, 1998), and on debates on cultural competence (Lau & Rodgers, 2021).

Researchers and practitioners have called for the development of new roles for health care staff (including ancillary workers), whereby recognition of the stress, memory problems and mental health needs of diverse refugee groups is crucial for effective primary health care workers such as nurses (Procter, 2006) and health visitors (Drennan & Joseph, 2005). In addition, there is a need for health services to develop and improve language and information services and close links with community-based organisations, specialist mental health services and services for survivors of torture and organised violence, as well as targeted health promotion and training of health workers (Feldman, 2006).

Moreover, a study by Ghebrehewet et al. (2002) has observed a range of difficulties for the delivery of appropriate health care for refugee and asylum seekers. These include a lack of information regarding the number of people seeking asylum, a lack of prior notification about arrival, shortfalls in additional health care resources, a lack of information about the health status of the people seeking asylum due to high mobility. Disabled asylum seekers are in a difficult position due to a lack of clear direction from policy makers, which exacerbates impoverished living due to a lack of service provision (Harris & Roberts, 2004).

From this research, taking into account the social context of asylum seekers and the difficulties in accessing services, some issues have been highlighted, such as: the need for information and support, the need for adequately qualified interpreters, as children often act as the main translators for their parents at medical appointments (Mountian, 2005), and the need for culturally sensitive approaches to health and mental health care.

Therefore, it is imperative that research and service providers take into account the social context of immigrants, asylum seekers and refugees, considering health and mental-health beliefs and attitudes. A perspective that encompasses the relation with broader cultural and social contexts considering the intersections between race, gender, class, age and disability can enlarge our understanding of mental health.

3.3 Immigration and health services in Brazil: gender, race and mental health

It is crucial to bear in mind that immigrants, refugees and asylum seekers do not form an homogenous group, in addition to the differences in service provision by host countries. Bureaucratic issues and a lack of structural resources for service provision may add further obstacles to settlement, as well as the way that immigration is socially conceived through intersections of gender, race, sexuality, class, disability and age. This sub-section based on the research conducted in Brazil ((*Otherness and migration: intersecting gender, race and class* (Mountian, 2015a) and *Intersectionality and otherness: trajectories of immigration and social network* (Appendix 1)) will investigate the impact of these social constraints on health and mental health practice.

The social and historical context in Brazil brings a number of issues to the fore, more specifically regarding how power relations in 'post-colonial' settings operate and resonate in everyday life. Current debates on post-colonial and decolonial studies (Mignolo, 2007; Quijano, 1992; Ballestrin, 2013) highlight the ongoing colonial heritage and how it contributes to the experience and configuration of subject positions, in this case, immigrants in Brazil.

Before turning to immigration and health services in Brazil, it is worthwhile considering some historical dimensions of the social context (for some further elements see Mountian & Gonzalez, 2019).[6] Brazil was colonised in 1500 led by the Portuguese Pedro Álvares Cabral. With an extractionist project, slavery first started with Indigenous people then with African people until abolition in 1888 (Ramos, 1997). Forced to work in plantations (sugarcane), mines (diamond) and in households, it was in this context that specific sexual and racial dynamics were established, together with moral and religious values. As Gilberto Freyre (1946) describes in *The Masters and The Slaves*, these relationships were based on the absolute hierarchical patriarchal-based power of the Master, who ruled and exerted control over his family (women and children) and slaves. This was done through an ambiguous and balanced equilibrium of dichotomies such as closeness and distance, and love and violence. The slavemaster's dynamic became, for Freyre (1946), the basis on which Brazilian society was established.

> The interplay of hierarchical social categories is foregrounded. On the one hand, the Portuguese slavemasters incorporated not only some of the habits of these enslaved peopled into their customs, affecting cultural practices, but also, and more crucially, they also incorporated into their households some of the offspring they had with enslaved women. The slavemaster held absolute power over white women, their children, and enslaved Black women and men. While this power was deemed to be absolute, in practice it lead to certain instances of accommodation, in strategies for slave survival that included, for instance, the acceptance of the incorporation of enslaved Black women into the masters' house as domestic slaves and at times as 'illicit' sexual partners. This planted the seed for the process of admixture and miscegenation that Freyre described as Brazil's defining characteristic. However, as Freyre points out, notwithstanding this incorporation, Portuguese male slavemasters maintained a hierarchical and extremely violent control over enslaved African women and men. This illustrates the importance of incorporating the temporal and local context of colonial relations into the analysis and application of intersectionality in the Brazilian context. We consider the importance of historical power relations in all contexts, because it enables an analysis of the inherent tensions and complex contradictions of subjugated subject positions. In short, inclusion of the colonial context in intersectionality pushes against a reductionist binary or hierarchical formulation.

The Catholic Church legitimised the position of slavemasters through the catechisation of Indigenous people by the Jesuits (Fausto, 1996). From 1808 to 1821, the Portuguese court moved to Brazil with the King Dom João VI, fleeing Napoleon's invasion, forming the United Kingdom of Portugal, Brazil and Algarves (from 1815). In 1822, Dom Pedro I, his son and regent prince declared independence from Portugal, founding the Empire of Brazil. In 1889 Brazil became a republic, although few people had the right to vote, excluding women and illiterate people. During this period, there was a State promotion of European immigration, as ex-enslaved Black people were seen as idle and indolent, not suited for paid labour, progressively disenfranchising them. Later immigration moved to the cities, particularly to the Southeast due to processes of industrialisation.

From 1930 to 1945 Getúlio Vargas governed Brazil with military support and dictatorship powers, then from 1951 to 1954 as elected president. From 1964 to 1985, Brazil was under military dictatorship. During the period of democratisation social movements (Feminist, Black, LGBTQI+ movements) could become more active and organised.

The impact of colonisation and slavery in contemporary Brazilian society is still seen, for example in the unequal socio-economic opportunities, and the lack of awareness of how sexism and racism is reproduced in society, as seen in the public polls[7] about the existence of racism in Brazil, or in debates on sexual and reproductive rights, which invisibilise and maintain this form of violence, also perpetuated through legislations.

> Inequality amongst intersectional social categories is seen in all levels in society. While Brazil has one of the strongest economies worldwide, the 7th largest in 2011 (IMF and IBGE), it is still marked by huge inequalities in terms of income and social welfare. In terms of GINI index parameters, Brazil stands for one of the 10 worst patterns of income distribution (0.549) among countries analyzed by PNUD (United Nations Programme for Development) in 2011 (Mountian, 2013b). Currently, Brazil has the highest rates of violence worldwide; the Ministry of Health reported 59.080 homicides in Brazil in the year of 2015 (Cerqueira et al., for IPEA & FBSP, 2017), particularly of Black people (Waiselfisz, 2016), and amongst these, of young, poor, Black males (Waiselfisz, 2011). Brazil is often cited as a country with the highest number of homicides of women (Waiselfisz, 2015) and transgender people (TGEU, 2016), followed by high incidence of violence against LGBTQI people, and violence and displacement of Indigenous people (CIMI, 2015).
>
> (Mountian & Gonzalez, 2019, p. 97)

These are important aspects to consider, particularly regarding how the colonial historical elements reflect in everyday life and reproduce specific power relations concerning 'Othering' processes.

Power and institutions

Taking into account these structural elements, I focus here on some dynamics of the encounters between immigrants and health services, showing how the categories of gender, race and sexuality operate within these encounters, which are often naturalised, invisibilised or stereotyped in discourse (Burman et al., 2004). The examples are based on the research projects conducted between 2012–2015 and 2015–2020, and the work with the Sao Paulo City Council project on health policy for migrants, aimed at sensitising health service providers on issues concerning the immigrant.

It is crucial here to highlight the difficulties stemming from institutional structural conditions and lack of resources. During the research, most professionals were engaged in service provision for immigrants, dealing with the lack of structural resources and creating and developing strategies for this population. These included outreach projects and using private mobile phones for translation, among others. The following critical analysis will focus on specific discourses reproduced within health care provision.

First, it is important to analyse how the signifier 'immigrant' operates, as a specific racial dynamic. 'Immigrants' were often considered Black people, coming from African Countries and Haiti, and Indigenous people, mostly from Bolivia and Peru. This discourse finds resonance with historical ideals surrounding desired European traits, reproducing a particular colonial discourse. It is noteworthy that the word 'gringo' or 'ex-patriate' is popularly used to designate Europeans and North Americans, or simply the country where they came from (e.g. American, German). These discursive differences point to the reproduction of hierarchical positions of immigrants, having an impact into the dynamics of 'racial' (in)visibility.

Second, health services presented a lack of structure and information regarding immigration, from the shortage of interpreters to deficits in knowledge regarding immigrant communities. In other services with a longer tradition in caring for immigrant populations however, profound expertise and an engagement with immigrant issues was observed, with these services coming to occupy an important role within the immigrant community. These are crucial aspects to consider in order to understand the lack of adherence to health treatments and access to health systems. Moreover, this lack of awareness of the immigration process can also create the possibility of naturalising exceptional circumstances, thereby risking hasty mental health diagnoses (Mountian & Rosa, 2015), as we will discuss further in the following sub-section.

Third, the presence of racist, xenophobic and sexist dynamics within health institutions is a constant challenge. The encounter between health services and immigrants brings these relations to the fore, as such beliefs may prevail, be it tacitly or not, within institutions. Therefore, it becomes crucial to interrogate the reproduction of common-sense discourses on immigrants (Simai & Baeninger, 2011) in health practice. In the research, such discourses were observed, for example, in the idea that immigrants bring disease, such as tuberculosis, to the country rather than considering the possibility of contracting the disease in overcrowded conditions in the host country. Tuberculosis has historically been associated with poverty and non-white populations since colonial times. Health professionals have observed that some of Bolivian immigrants, for example, live in inadequate accommodation and work in overcrowded sweatshops in precarious conditions that do not meet labour law requirements, in some cases in a situation tantamount to slave labour.

Awareness of the informal labour conditions in sweatshops, the dynamics of trans-immigration, more specifically in keeping relations with the country of departure and survival strategies (and of the family) in both countries (Freitas, 2013), are important to consider. In this sense, Freitas considers Tarrius' notion of circular territory (*territórios circulares*, Tarrius), as made up of groups characterised by shared experience of same conditions of displacement (2013).

This discursive re-enactment of colonial working conditions intersects with race, gender and class, which can be seen in this case, for example, when Bolivian mothers are blamed for their children's health, while their working and living conditions and the lack of accessible childcare are often overlooked. This gendered and racialised discourse is contrasted with an idealised image of motherhood, oblivious to wider social conditions. Feminist researchers (Phoenix, 2011) claim that transnational motherhood is a feminist issue, as it is often the mother (not the father) who is subject to criticism for not taking sufficient care of their children, when they are far from their children due to immigration, or as in this case, when they are with their children. This foregrounds a number of issues regarding 'mothering on the margins' (Phoenix, 2011), characterised as a 'non-normative' motherhood, wherein they are subject to public censure.

Craig and O'Dell (2011) analyse the discursive production of 'Othered' mothers, outside the idealised forms of motherhood, predominantly based on a Western white bourgeois ideal. They argue that not accounting for these differences can widen the disjunction between dominant discourses on motherhood and the social context of women, (re)producing the othering position of immigrant women in discourse.

It is crucial to consider the position of women in the family and nation, as the moral, emotional and economic responsibility for maintaining the family often falls on their shoulders. Phoenix (2011) highlights that transnational families must negotiate circuits of emotion, material goods and financial support. Citing the term 'emotional transnationalism' from Wolf (2002), Phoenix argues that emotions are defined through migration and separation, as the emotional and economic work across borders falls to women. The experience of serial migration, that is, when the family members migrate at different times, produces separation of mothers and children, who do not have the resources to migrate together (Phoenix & Seu, 2013). In this context, mothers more often than fathers participate in 'global care chains' (Parreñas, 2005 *apud* Phoenix &

Seu, 2013), requiring the development of diverse strategies for mothering and 'emotional transnationalism' (Phoenix & Seu, 2013).

When analysing the relationship between gender and immigration, it is vital to consider the roles attributed to women in the family, particularly concerning for care and support, are important to be accounted in the analysis of gender and immigration, which continue after settlement. Moreover, it is important to highlight the risks of sexual and domestic violence and the increase of sexually transmitted diseases among women who might be working in precarious conditions, with little access to health services (Teles, 2007).

Another aspect that is relevant to highlight regards discourses surrounding 'cultural differences'. In our research discourses on 'cultural differences', race and gender operated in the narrative that Latin American women (not including Brazilian women), particularly from Bolivia, are more submissive than Brazilian women. It is important to contextualise the so-called 'submission' of women in patriarchal societies, requiring a critical analysis of the position of women in these relationships. Moreover, how discourses on cultural differences appear here, can seem to imply that 'they' are not as 'modern' as 'us' (McClintock, 1995), which can reproduce specific colonial discourses in a patriarchal context. Further, it is relevant to highlight that in this case, some health service providers developed strategies to listen to women alone, without the company of any male companion, as many women arrived accompanied by men, and did not feel safe to comfortable talking about their issues in front of them.

Moreover, service providers reported that some Muslim women preferred to be seen by female doctors, a request that was also be observed in members of other religious groups. This once again highlights the relevance of investigating the intersections between gender, religion, race and culture in relation to health care provision.

Fourth, sexuality and its dynamics in immigration and settlement are often overlooked. LGBTQI+phobia has an important impact into the processes of influence on international and domestic immigration processes, as some people have to flee their countries due to persecution stemming from their sexual identity and practices, a situation also observed in some contexts in Brazil (Mountian, 2015b). The recognition of the effects of LGBTQI+phobia is crucial understanding immigration and settlement processes and to provide an adequate listening and environment and listening in health institutions (further discussed in Chapter 4).

Discourses that place migrants in particularly vulnerable positions can obscure their histories and everyday struggles, bringing to the fore the importance of interrogating these power relations, in order to create possibilities for other discursive positions. From this research and in other contexts (Mountian, 2007, 2015, 2020), the importance of migrants' rights to health services and other institutional and government assistance has been highlighted, which can create networks and spaces of support, that can enable different discursive positions.

3.4 Reflections on the encounter: decolonising mental health

In this sub-section, I focus on the analysis of the encounter between psy-disciplines and immigrants. The work with immigrants (as well as other culturally diverse groups, such as religious fundamentalist communities) presents a number of challenges, not only involving language but also to culture, which, while they outline a space for rethinking strategies, they crucially interrogate 'our' own psy-culture. Two main aspects are emphasised here: first regarding the risks of hasty diagnosis of mental health diagnoses and over-prescription of psychiatric medications, and second, regarding the acknowledgement of how assumptions of mental health and health are culturally located.

In previous research in England and in Brazil (Mountian, 2005, 2007, 2020), a number of issues were raised by immigrants and health professionals, such as the difficulties in accessing health services (Mountian, 2007), the lack of adherence to treatment (Mountian, 2015b, 2020) and concerns about the over-prescription of anti-depressants, particularly for women (Mountian, 2005). These examples put into question the encounter with the 'Othered' immigrant and, crucially, required a critical analysis of taken-for-granted views on tacitly assumed understandings within health and mental health.

It is crucial, therefore, to question how gender, class, 'race', age and 'culture' (among other categories) are framed within these discursive practices. Drawing on the 'normalised absence and pathologised presence' of specific groups (Phoenix, 1987), it illustrates the experiences of asylum seekers and refugees in health care provision environments. The pathologised presence of asylum seekers and refugees in health care services requires further careful analysis, particularly when exceptional circumstances (war, famine, settlement) overlapping with intersectional categories are assumed to be essential characteristics of the immigrant, rather than being understood as circumstances that the individual is subjected to, as such, mental illness is normalised, upholding an individualising view on. This creates a situation wherein mental health issues become naturalised, reifying an individualistic conception of mental health, which downplays the external conditions as relevant to the formation of pathological conditions.

A critical analysis on the diagnoses of depression provides some insights into this dynamic. First, there is the risk of understanding depression as a 'natural' condition, rather than as the outcome of exceptional events, structural vulnerability, racism, sexism and pre and post-migratory processes. Second, considering the circumstances of asylum seekers such as, delays in the asylum-seeking process, impossibility to work, lack of information, uncertainties, racism and sexism (Fang et al., 2015; Mountian, 2015b, 2020), depression can be seen as a 'response' to the inadequate living conditions. Third, the administration of anti-depressants without any other additional support can operate in a way that end up silencing those who are not currently participating in any formal social mechanisms of social inclusion.

Fourth, over-prescription of anti-depressants for women is also observed among asylum seekers and refugees (Dawson, 2003), and how this affects the care of the family, involves other facets of gender differentiation.

On culture

> It is important to further analyse the way discourses on 'culture' appear in relation to immigrants. When 'culture' operates as a way to undervalue or separate the subject, placed as the Other in discourse, it acts as a form of neo-racism, displacing discourses from 'race' to 'culture'. 'Culture' is commonly used with a specific meaning, encompassing people from a specific geographic area, however, people from the same geographic area might not share similar values (e.g. social and political backgrounds, race, class, gender, religion, language). Culture, therefore, is not a fixed term (Brah, 1996) and must also be considered in relation to the local culture, as such, the way that culture is constituted within the encounters must also be interrogated.
>
> The interplay between gender and culture was seen through the othered position of immigrant women and motherhood at the margins, particularly in the social control of mothers during transnational migration, and in discourses on immigrant women as more submissive, which can carry an implied idea that 'our' culture is not gender divided. Recognising the vulnerabilities in which women and LGBTQI+ people are circumscribed is paramount for the development of services.

Uncovering these dynamics is crucial to recognising the intrinsic views and power relations in which the immigrant is embedded, as also claimed by LGBTQI+ communities, Black and Ethnic Minority Community Services, and to acknowledge the situatedness of the psy-culture. This is particularly important for a decolonised practice towards minoritised groups, bringing to the fore the need to recognise the social context of both the subject and the views on psychology and psychiatry.

Health service providers with experience of working with diverse groups argue for the need to consider migrants' views on health and mental health and to incorporate these perspectives into work with immigrants. I highlight some of the examples from the research (Appendix 1) here. First, the importance of taking into account differences in understanding of health care, including the use of different forms of medication. Second, the challenges of working with religious fundamentalist groups and negotiating medical and religious practices for health treatment (e.g. HIV treatment). Third, in situations of domestic violence, some health units developed strategies to support women without the presence of men. Fourth, in the context of the pandemic, some providers also argued for the value of learning from migrant communities that had already experienced epidemics (Mountian et al., 2020). From the research on drug use and asylum seekers in the UK, there was little evidence of drug use in the immigrant groups interviewed (mostly religious). However, drug education is still an important strategy, considering advocacy and outreach services for groups that cannot easily access health services.

A need for adequate interpreters was reported in all studies, as well as a need for awareness of the experiences and challenges immigrants, refugees and asylum seekers face, including racism, sexism, LGBTQI+phobia and xenophobic violence. A multi-racial work force was suggested as an effective strategy. Finally, it is highlighted that the active participation of migrants in dialogue with health service providers is important for the development of health services (Mountian, 2016) and policy making (Bacron, 2021).

Final remarks

This chapter highlighted the importance of considering power relations in our analysis, including the historical dynamics of discourses and how these are active in the (in)visibility of specific groups. This foregrounds the importance of an ongoing posture of reflexivity from service providers in their work with Othered groups, challenging the discursive reproduction of the position of the Other in everyday life and in service provision, so as to provide space for other encounters.

The main issues highlighted refer to considering the subject and the social context of immigration into account for the development of health interventions. The analysis of the intersections between gender, sexuality, race, class and age showed the specificities of these groups and the need to engage in these. The analysis points out to a culturally situated medical view on health and how the encounter with diverse groups can allow for different forms of understanding health.

Notes

1. Scalabrine and Pastoral support for immigrants (Costa, 2011; Russo, 2011)
2. Early intervention and outreach should be creative, advertising should be done in diverse formats, posters should be written in different languages, young asylum seekers could participate more actively in early intervention (e.g. making posters), young asylum seekers are not aware of drug services, confidentiality arrangements should be made clear and parents should also be aware about drugs in the areas where they live and should give consent for drug education. Furthermore, there is a need for more training for service providers on issues related to drugs.
3. Male, 41 years old, refugee from Iraq
4. Male, 46 years old, asylum seeker from Somalia
5. Male, Somali
6. Parts of this sub-section is based on the chapter: Mountian, I. and Gonzalez, E.C. (2019). "Reflections on the theory and practice of intersectionality: immigration and health provision services in Brazil", p.92–104. In Nayak, S. and Robbins, R. (eds). Intersectionality in Social Work: activism and practice in context. London: Routledge
7. See http://csbh.fpabramo.org.br/o-que-fazemos/editora/teoria-e-debate/edicoes-anteriores/sociedade-discriminacao-racial-e-preconceit and http://congressoemfoco.uol.com.br/noticias/vox-populi-82-da-populacao-e-contra-aborto/

4 Mental health and sexuality

Reflections on older *travestis* and transwomen in Brazil

This chapter follows the debate on the situated understandings of gender and sexuality and the impact on medical practice and the theory of health and mental health. This analysis, drawing on critical perspectives on LGBTTTQIA+ and mental health, will centre on studies with trans people. These debates are based on the research conducted in 2012 with older *travestis* and transsexual women in Brazil and on the research on trans people's access to education in 2013.

For our analysis, it is fundamental to contextualise the position of *travestis* and trans people in society, and how this impacts health and mental health perspectives. Three main aspects are highlighted here: first, the effects of pathologisation on trans people, given the historical views of transsexuality and homosexuality as a mental illness in psychiatry. This is a key issue, emphasising how othering processes figure in the medical science and practice, as discussed in Chapter 2. Second, discrimination against LGBTQI+ people when present in health services becomes an obstacle to accessing medical and psychological care. Discrimination also becomes a hindrance to accessing education, employment and housing. Third, from the research with elderly transwomen and *travestis* in Brazil, the need to consider the specificities of these groups becomes evident, taking into consideration intersections of gender, race, class, age and disability, in health services and public policy.

4.1 Contextualising *travestis* and trans people in Brazil

This section presents some aspects of the social context of trans people in Brazil, based on the report *A critical analysis of public policies on education and LGBT rights in Brazil* (Mountian, 2014a). The study on access to education of transgender people in Brazil was commissioned by the Institute of Development Studies at the University of Sussex, coordinated by Ilana Mountian, supervised by Marco Aurelio Prado and Sonia Correa, and fieldwork undertaken by Igor Monteiro and Rodrigo Alencar. The research interviewed educators, LGBTQI+ activists and education policy makers, and assessed education policies for LGBTQI+ people and poverty in Brazil.

DOI: 10.4324/9780429263415-7

In the past two decades, up to 2018, there were some important improvements regarding poverty reduction, although the number of people living in extreme poverty is still high.[1] From 1992 to 2012, around 12 million people were no longer living in absolute poverty, a reduction from 13.7% (in 1992) to 3.6% (2012) (IPEA, 2013). However, it is important to highlight that social inequality is still profoundly marked.

> If you apply the Gini coefficient to measure income inequality, in 2011, Brazil achieved the lowest level of inequality since 1960, the first year this measurement was used. Between 1960 and 1990, inequality grew from 0.5367 to 0.6091. From that point it decreased until 2010, when it reached 0.5304. It continued to fall in 2011, when it reached the lowest number ever, 0.527. Even though the inequality coefficient was at its lowest ever two years ago, Brazil continues to be one of the 12 most unequal countries in the world.
>
> (Soares, 2013)

Data on discrimination and violence against LGBTQI+ people is still scarce in Brazil; however, reports seem to indicate high levels of discrimination. CLAM (Latin American Center for Sexuality and Human Rights) in the study on the LGBTQI+ Parades in Sao Paulo, Rio de Janeiro and Recife from 2003 to 2006 reported that discrimination was mostly experienced in families, communities and educational environments. In a nationwide survey (2014 subjects) in 2009 the Perseu Abramo Foundation found that 90% of interviewees believed that there is prejudice against LGBTQI+ people. Significantly, only 28% of interviewees admitted to having discriminated against LGBTQIA+ people.

The Gay Group from Bahia (GGB) through analysis of press reports on assassinations of LGBT+ people identified more than 300 murders in 2021, an increase of 8% compared to 2021, 51% were gay men and 37% travestis and transwomen. Unsurprisingly, Brazil has been identified as a worldwide hotspot of homophobic and transphobic crimes (TGEU, 2013). Benevides and Nogueira (2021) reported that in 2020 there were 175 homicides of trans people and an increase in violence, attempts of murder and suicide. Moreover, the sub-notification of cases has to be considered, particularly for transmen (Pfeil & Alves, 2024). Benevides and Nogueira (2021) highlight the lack of appropriate policies and the effects of the persecution from conservative governmental sectors and campaigns against LGBTQIA+ people.

Illiteracy, as one indicator correlated with poverty (Mountian, 2014a), showed an important improvement, dropping significantly over the last 30 years, with around 7.9% of the population over 10 years of age remaining illiterate, corresponding to 13.1 million people (IBGE, PNAD, 2011, p. 109, 110). In 2001, social development programmes including *Bolsa Família* identified 5.1 million completely illiterate people among its beneficiaries, and

9.4 million functionally illiterate individuals (few years of education), which shows a correlation between poverty and access to education.

The impact of LGBTphobia on education can hinder access to education for this population. A number of studies have observed discrimination against LGBTQIA+ people in schools. A study by Castro et al. (2004) demonstrated that 25% of students interviewed (16,500) did not want to have a homosexual colleague. Another study funded by the Ministry of Education and conducted by FIPE10 (Mazzon, 2009) with 15,000 students in 501 schools reported a wide range of acts of humiliation and homophobic violence in public schools. Souza et al. (2012), in a study in the state of Pernambuco with 110 *travestis* in the cities of Recife and Olinda, showed that 44.9% did not finish secondary school (*ensino médio*) and 79.2% left their parental home before the age of 18 due to their gender identity and sexual orientation, also seen in prior research (Mountian, 2013b), which is a crucial aspect regarding vulnerability.

> We can say that there are numerous situations in which schools deny the existence of this population [*travestis* and transsexual people]. Some trans people left school, some survived prejudice and managed to do something by themselves, to attend a university and to work in areas of public education and health. . . . But there are few people who managed to do this. We have around 60 teachers who are trans people in Brazil. I believe that there can be more but many are afraid to come out and suffer transphobia.
>
> (Interviewee public administrator, teacher)

Policies to tackle sexual discrimination in schools were initiated in the 1990s, with strong resistance from conservative sectors. These initiatives cannot be entirely disconnected from the Brazilian response to HIV/AIDS, combating discrimination against LGBTQIA+ people and sex workers (Parker, 2003; Galvão, 2002). From 2003 to 2010 there were a series of federal guidelines (under the Worker's Party government) focused on the rights and needs of LGBTQI+ people, also seen as a result of LGBTQI+ activism. The 2004 programme Brazil Without Homophobia (*Brasil sem Homofobia*), considered a key turning point, covered a number of policy areas such as health, education, labour, human rights and public security. The programme was run by the National Centre for LGBT Rights (*Coordenação Geral de Promoção dos Direitos LGBT*), located at the Special Secretary for Human Rights. In 2008, the programme guidelines were defined by the National Plan for LGBT Citizenship (*Plano de Cidadania LGBT – Plano Nacional de Promoção da Cidadania e Direitos Humanos de LGBT – Lésbicas, Gays, Bissexuais, Travestis e Transexuais*) and were approved at the First Conference on LGBT Policies, which included several education policy resolutions (Mountian, 2014a).

Studies (Mello et al., 2012; Mountian, 2014a) have observed a number of obstacles and impediments to the implementation of policies to combat discrimination against LGBTQIA+ people in the education system, which has a direct impact on social inequality. The development and implementation of education policies against discrimination of LGBTQIA+ people (Junqueira, 2009) in schools is crucial, including as part of a wider agenda that understands sexuality and gender beyond stereotypical perspectives and considers the intersections between race, class, age, disability, religion, regional specificities and others. These policies must work as an integrated and coordinated multi-disciplinary strategy to overcome exclusion, social inequality and poverty.

4.2 *Travestis*, transgender, transsexual women and ageing

From this social contextualisation of trans people in Brazil, I raise some key questions that emerged from the research '*Travestis*, transsexual women and Ageing' (2012),[2] coordinated by Ilana Mountian and with fieldwork undertaken by Liliane Anderson, Igor Monteiro, Frederico Viana Machado and Rafaela Vasconcelos. This study was part of the research partnership 'The visibility of gendered bodies and their political and everyday implications' (*A visibilidade de corpos gendrados e seus desdobramentos políticos e cotidianos*), funded by CNPQ, with Universidade Federal de Minas Gerais, Universidade Federal do Estado de Sao Paulo, Universidade Federal da Bahia and Universidade Federal de Pernambuco. For this qualitative research, we interviewed *travestis* considered elderly (N-5), who highlighted a number of crucial issues regarding health, immigration, body and history. The interviews were conducted by a *travesti*, two cisgender women and two cisgender men.

The interviewees, all over 46 years old, were from diverse parts of Brazil. Four of them are black and all came from families of less privileged social classes, from a city in Bahia (N-1), a city in Minas Gerais (N-1), Belo Horizonte, the capital of Minas Gerais (N-1) and Rio de Janeiro city (N-1) and Sao Paulo city (N-1). Four interviewees had experience of national and international migration processes. Currently, they work in different professions (hairdressers, singers, prostitutes), while some are activists for the recognition and defence of human rights and citizenship for *travestis*, transwomen and transmen.

Transphobia in Brazil has been reported in various sectors (Amaral et al., 2014; Transgender Europe, 2016, 2023). The understanding of how the dynamics and effects of transphobia and homophobia operate in different contexts is fundamental, as well as taking regional specificities and the intersections of social categories of race, sexuality, class, age and disability into account. While the interviewees highlighted issues that arose within local contexts, at the same time, they emphasise elements that traverse experiences common to diverse locations in Brazil, particularly regarding the effects of exclusion.

In this chapter, I will privilege the voices of the participants (Browne & Nash, 2010), through excerpts from the interviews, in which interviewees highlighted crucial issues for consideration regarding health, mental health and otherness. The main themes raised in the interviews were related to the need to account for the specificities of this population for the development of research and public policy, the importance of intersectionality (gender, race, class, disability and age) and, crucially, how transphobia as structural violence permeates the trajectories, stories and experiences of *travestis*, transwomen, transmen and trans masculinities.

Throughout the interviews it could be observed how interviewees traced a historical biographical narrative in relation to their context, recounting transphobic and homophobic violence and offering testimony of political and social changes in Brazil. The participants highlighted issues related to their sexuality and ageing, their relationship with their own body, access to health services, safety and possibilities for employment and social inclusion. These aspects are fundamental to understanding the experiences of *travestis* and transwomen, underlining the need for further research, and public policies that take this population into account.

Moreover, the themes of transsexuality and immigration, as well as studies on the intersection between ageing and sexuality, remain little explored in the field of psychology, although there is growth in studies of transsexuality in recent years (Amaral et al., 2014; Nardi et al., 2013), research on ageing of *travestis*, transsexual women and trans men (Antunes, 2010; Fernandes et al., 2015; Kimmel, 2014; Siverskog, 2014), on the sexuality of transgender populations in old age (Bauer et al., 2013; Witten, 2015) and on studies on transsexuality and race (Graham et al., 2014). The present chapter provides contributions to the area and emphasises the importance of giving voice to these groups. It is relevant to note the importance of social movements for the visibility and struggle for citizenship and human rights for these communities (Prado et al., 2010; Facchini et al., 2020), such as ANTRA (*Associação Nacional de Travestis e Transsexuais, Brazilian Travesti and Transsexual Association*) and IBRAT (Instituto Brasileiro de Transmasculinidades) and the international movements against transpathologisation, which have gradually advanced the cause of trans rights in Brazil, Europe, the USA, Canada and others (Tosh, 2016; Benevides, 2023).

Transphobia and trans identification

> Most *travestis* are marginal all their lives and when they get old, they become old marginals (*marginais*).
>
> (Interviewee no 1, 08 February 2012)[3]

Travesti is a gender identity from Brazil and other Latin American countries. This quote highlights the social position of *travestis* and transgender women in Brazil, foregrounding important issues to consider in the experience of *travestis*, that is, of being on the margins of society in a specific way, as the word marginal in Portuguese used in everyday language also denotes a moral judgement of the individual as 'no good', outcast and scum.

Taking up Spivak's (1988) reflections on the impossibilities of the subaltern to speak and to be heard, having their voice always mediated, we interrogate how can the *travesti* speak. In this marginal discursive position, through fetichised social relations, the subject is often objectified, viewed as the Other and often characterised as a homogeneous Other. This abject (Butler, 1999) discursive position reifies the subject, preventing us from considering them as subjects with desire or agency. In this sense, the subaltern is seen as not participating in the dialogical possibilities of speech (to represent meaning, to perform and to speak) and of self-representation. Rather they are spoken about or spoken for. As such 'the subject is not seen as a representative consciousness (one re-presenting reality adequately). These two senses of representation – within state formation and the law, on the one hand, and in subject-predication, on the other – are related but irreducibly discontinuous' (Spivak, 1988/2011, p. 70).

The trans body calls the rigidity of gender performances into question, challenging what is historically conceived as biological and transgressing codes of gender norms, which vary according to local understandings of gender. The trans body makes clear discourses on cisgenderism, of what is socially expected from cisgender women and men, while the non-acceptance of *travestis* in society is continuously reiterated.

Notably, prevalent discourses about *travesti*s and transsexual women are still permeated by moral-religious and medical discourses (Amaral et al., 2014). *Travestis* are placed in a challenging position not only due to binary sex divisions but also in relation to traditional forms of gender identity. The attempt to homogenise gender identities and social categories proved to be an impossibility. However, we can highlight some common characteristics that pervade various localities within patriarchal and cisgender societies, more precisely regarding the power dynamics stemming from cisgender and heterosexual social norms. While we certainly cannot affirm in a general fashion the exclusion and oppression of all subjects, we can argue that subjects who do not fulfil expected gender and sexual norms can suffer some form of oppression (Butler, 1999/2008), crucially, considering the way dynamics of intersectional categories of race, class, age and disability operate in specific contexts (Burman, 2010; Chantler, 2007; McClintock, 1995; Pisciteli, 2008), within heterosexual, cisgender and colonial social perspectives.

This travesti identity is recognised in parts of Latin America, and in Brazil, marking the first wave of the non-cisgender movement in the struggle for rights, the travesti movement (Benevides, 2020). Traditionally *Travestis* in Brazil often experience social exclusion, many coming from economically and socially disadvantaged classes, having experienced racist and sexist violence, with limited opportunities for inclusion into the labour market and many working as sex workers. As Kulick (1998, p. 7) describes:

> In most cities, including Salvador, *travestis* are so discriminated against that many of them avoid venturing out onto the street during the day. They are regularly the victims of violent police brutality and random assassinations. Most of them come from very poor backgrounds and many remain poor throughout their lives, living a hand-to-mouth existence and dying before the age of fifty from violence, drug abuse, health problems caused by the silicone they inject into their bodies, or, increasingly, AIDS.

The history of *travestility* in Brazil shows how this identity was marginalised, often associated with prostitution and vulnerability. The *travesti* identity was often used as an overarching identity category in the broad spectrum of trans and queer identities (Hutta & Balzer, 2013). Contemporary debates highlight the need for other identifications and, crucially, also for the importance of affirming the position of *travesti*, as a political identity position engaged in resistance and activism. In the case of this research, all participants identified themselves as *travesti*s and affirmed this identity positively, referring to being *travesti* as a sexual political identity. It is also noteworthy that one of the interviewees adopted a male name and used the grammatical male gender to talk about 'himself' while maintaining the self-identification of *travesti*. We highlight here, therefore, the importance of considering the self-identification of *travestis*, as well as transsexual and transgender women and transmen, seen here as a political position in identity politics.

> There is no definition in my humble opinion (it even rhymed). For me, being and identifying as *travesti* besides reinforcing a political identity, is a state of mind that has been with me since I can remember, obviously there are many complexities in this debate and I consider most of them.
>
> (Keila Simpson, 2021, Social media, Keila Simpson is the founder of the Associação Nacional de Travestis e Transsexuais)[4]

Vartabedian (2014a) traces this debate in academic studies, pointing out that the notion of 'third gender', developed in the 1980s, was not incorporated into the traditional gender dichotomies. In the 1990s, the term 'transgender' is highlighted as a distinct possibility for the political and theoretical referents of sexual diversity, and self-affirmation. However, the attempts at institutionalising the term 'transgender' as an overarching form of incorporating all non-normative identities can homogenise experiences and risks excluding specific groups, as not all *travestis* and transexual and transvestite individuals refer to themselves as transgender (Vartabedian, 2014a), a nuance that can be elided within the term 'transgender' (Vicente,

2021). Therefore, it is necessary to consider the specificities of each self-identified group according to the social context, that is, considering the plurality of experiences, economic vulnerabilities and gender binary transgressions involved (Drager & Platero, 2021).

In the Brazilian context, the debate about the differences between *travestis* and transsexuals can occur in everyday situations, although these do not define the difference between these identities. In some specific contexts, a higher status may be implied. In the study by Silva et al. (2019), differences were found in terms of social class, particularly with regard to the possibility of working outside prostitution, which reduces the risk of homicide. Nevertheless, transphobia is present in all cases. Those most at risk of homicide are those who have not undergone gender reassignment surgery, so that conforming to gender norms would increase their safety and likelihood of survival, which also intersects with categories of race and class.

It is therefore important to take the social context into consideration when looking at the specificities of the communities and their demands, as well as the formation of political identities (Motta, 2004). Moreover, as already discussed, these representations and political identities should not reduce the identifications of the individual or essentialise them (Butler, 1999/2008). *Travesti* is seen simultaneously as a political identity, self-identification and form of life experience rather than as a homogeneous category, in face of the multiplicity of experience (Siqueira, 2004) and social recognition. *Travesti*s are considered, therefore, to be all those who self-identify as *travesti*s.

Transphobia and ageing

This chapter outlines some dimensions that characterise the everyday experience of *travesti*s and many transsexual and transgender women, given that gender non-conforming populations frequently share experiences of various forms of oppression, exclusion and violence, often being denied access to basic human rights (education, health, safety, work, housing).

> I see that today the *travesti* lives the night very intensely, as if it was the last night of her life, because she doesn't know if she will survive the next day or if she will wake up dead somewhere. So, it is as if she is living the last day of her life.
>
> (Interviewee 1, 8 February 2012)

Within this context, the experiences of ageing of this population have to be carefully investigated. There is a lack of research that focuses on the ageing of transgender, transsexual people and *travesti*s, as well as in LGBTQI+ studies in general (Alves, 2010; Simões, 2011). By disregarding age, research runs the risk of assuming a particular 'productive' notion of subject. Discourses on the 'normal' subject refer to those with an agile body, who are fully able and efficient in their functions, consonant with the view of youth as a stage marked by 'dynamism and creativity' (Debert, 2010, p. 51). As Pocahy (2014, p. 225) argues in his research on men who have sex with older men:

> Some performances of gender and sexuality are only made possible through a discourse on age, imposing what is right or wrong for each phase of life. Therefore, it seems strategic to investigate how age creates conditions of intelligibility and how it articulates with gender and sexuality in the face of the biopolitical project of Western societies.

In the case of older heterosexual cisgender women, sexuality is often seen as an infringement, at times a taboo, revealing the traditional interdictions on female sexuality, which is frequently understood as promiscuous, uncontrollable and dangerous, and therefore as requiring control. In this context, women and particularly older women are given the role of representative and guardian of the nation's morality (McClintock, 1995; Yuval-Davis, 1997). Alves (2010, p. 217) in their research on female homosexuality and ageing points out that:

> The idea that aged bodies have no space in the erotic market is widespread and this disadvantage ends up keeping older people away from the exercise of sexual conquest. This image is even stronger when it comes to women. As they get older, women are seen and see themselves as sexually unattractive. The body marks of ageing, such as wrinkles and white hair, are devalued from the aesthetic point of view and compromise the seductive potential of that body (Goldenberg, 2008). It is also stated that in Brazil this aesthetic devaluation of the older body is quite widespread, reflected in the high number of people who undergo (or would like to undergo) various procedures, including surgical, that promise physical rejuvenation.[5]

In the case of *travestis*, transwomen and transmen it is relevant to consider how these discursive elements of interdiction and control regulate the body. What are the discursive possibilities for older *travestis*? There are several questions that are pertinent for us here. First, it is fundamental to consider the social exclusion that marks the lives of *travestis* and transwomen and transmen, and second, it is necessary to consider the issues related to self-image, body interventions and possibilities for social inclusion, including employment, particularly affecting black *travestis* (Hutta & Balzer, 2013). Regarding social exclusion, authors highlight the abject position in which they find themselves, since they are not recognised in the frames of intelligibility of sexual norms (Miskolci, 2009 *apud* Antunes, 2010; Fernandes et al., 2015). In this sense, Antunes and Mercadante (2011) argue that the elderly *travestis* are 'accused of putting at risk the flow considered correct. For this reason, they are targeted, surveilled, watched, classified, excluded and subjected to treatment for correction'. Thus, the 'transgression' of social bodily and identity norms places them in a vulnerable social position, leading to their repeated exclusion.

Given the social marginalisation experienced by this community, the lack of research and national statistical data on the life expectancy for *travestis*, transwomen and transmen is notable. Anecdotal reports appear to point towards a low life expectancy for *travesti*s (some say around 40 years old), a fact that may reflect the risk and vulnerability of *travesti*s and transwomen in extremely transphobic contexts. Data relating to trans population homicide rates places Brazil as the country with the highest rate worldwide (TGEU, 2014: Benevides & Bonfim, 2021), subject to physical and psychological violence, high rates of self-harm associated or not with attempted suicide (Rodrigues & Magri, 2021, Sao Paulo monitoring project). In 2022, it was registered 131 trans people murdered (Benevides, 2023).

Black and poor individuals and those working in prostitution are at highest risk of homicide, which Silva et al. (2019) describes as 'transnecropolítica'. Early deaths associated with contamination from HIV, health complications resulting from body modifications (often performed informally), the risks and vulnerabilities arising from precarious living conditions (e.g. living on the streets and in shelters) (Rodrigues et al., 2021 – Sao Paulo Monitoring) and difficulties associated with accessing health services should also be considered. Death certificates frequently adopt the birth name, not respecting the individual's *travesti* or trans woman identity (Silva et al., 2019).

Moreover, it is also relevant to investigate the possibility for older *travesti*s to be present in public spaces, or more precisely, their frequent invisibility in public spaces. In this sense, it is pertinent to highlight the perception of ageing, since *travestis* are already considered elderly at the age of 40, which is correlated with their life expectancy. In this context, authors (Antunes, 2010; Siqueira, 2004) emphasise the importance for *travestis* to reach old age with dignity.

> It was not enough to be treated as a 'lady' ('*senhora*') on the street, it was not enough to be shown to the ladies' room or to be offered a seat on the bus, it is necessary to be a successful lady, in the sense of having 'escaped' AIDS, dependency on drugs, of being able to move around in different social strata, to be respected where you live and to be a wealthy lady (*senhora de posses*).
>
> (Siqueira, 2009, p. 44)[6]

Being recognised as a 'lady' is an important aspect for some *travesti*s. Antunes (2010) in his research highlights that interviewees felt satisfied when they were seen as 'ladies', which at times can also be a status before their community and society at large. For Siqueira (2009), being viewed as a 'lady' compensates the loss of social status linked to old age. Ageing for *travestis* was mentioned as another dimension contributing to their social exclusion:

> They think they're going to stay young for the rest of their lives. If a young *travesti* already has many problems, imagine an old one, it

> will be much more difficult, because you are called various things, old, 'faggot' (*maricona*). The young ones look at us and say: 'you are old, nobody wants you anymore!'
>
> (Interviewee No. 1, February 8, 2012)

This extract highlights how ageing is seen as unpleasant and undesirable, adding another layer of social exclusion.

Health and body

The ageing of *travestis* and transwomen has its specificities, affecting bodily changes and possibilities for social inclusion. The interviewees narrate the changes related to their bodily transformations and the difficulties of accessing health services:

> The *travesti*, when she gets old will have more problems than any other person because of the excess of hormones she took and for having applied silicone, her health will be weaker. She knows that she needs to see a doctor, but when she gets there, she will be victim of mockery and ridicule, they will make a point of calling her, very loudly, by her male name. So, she won't go to the doctor, and this is a right of any human being, in addition to leisure and security.
>
> (Interviewee 1, February 8, 2012)

The difficulties in accessing health services in health institutions due to transphobia were highlighted, as well as how services and public policy were unable to account for the specificities of the trans population (as seen also in other studies, Bicev & Aprile, 2021; Crenitte, 2021). Bodily changes are an important aspect for many *travestis,* as outlined by Pelúcio (2005):

> It is a process that never ends. Building a body and taking care of it is one of the major concerns of *travestis*. They are always seeking 'perfection', which means 'looking like a woman' ('*passar por mulher*'), a beautiful and desirable woman, usually 'white' and bourgeois. In search of this image, they refine their features, tan their bodies, adorn themselves with clothes that resemble glamorous women, choose names of actresses and Hollywood muses or pop singers.[7]
>
> (Pelúcio, 2005 *apud* Nogueira & León, 2012, p. 59)

For this process, a series of bodily interventions are often performed, such as the use of hormones, and application of industrial silicone and implants, among others. In Brazil, these procedures are very expensive, and there are long waiting lists to carry them out in the public health system, among other obstacles, leaving this population more vulnerable when they perform these interventions in informal ways (Mountian et al., 2012). The effects of these procedures on older bodies are relevant for consideration by health services.

The difficulties in accessing health services and the importance of accounting for the specificities of trans people are fundamental aspects highlighted in the research.

Work and ageing

The ageing of trans people was also highlighted in relation to the (im)possibility of finding employment. As already noted, the very idea of ageing differs for transwomen, such that many *travesti*s are already considered 'old' by 40, an age that refers to social perception of the body and its transformations, but also depending on what the market demands of them (such as sex work). The interviewees reported difficulties in finding employment, and within this transphobic context, it was observed that some *travesti*s 'begin to masculinise' for labour inclusion.

> How am I going to have money to support myself? I don't have any income, I don't have any savings, I don't have anything. I think that it is necessary to begin to observe these things, that I think that it is precisely these questions that will be asked, that we will try to understand and what to do to help this population. Perhaps this is why *travesti*s in Brazil begin to masculinize when they turn fifty, sixty, precisely to be able to go back into society as a person, which they could do very well being a *travesti*. (Interviewee 2, February 27, 2012).
>
> The great majority, and some that I could observe, is that when they get to this age, the advanced age, they first start to give up their identity. They start to worship more the male appearance. This is terrible. This happens a lot here in Brazil. In Europe we don't observe this, we see that in Europe transwomen continue even when they are old, but as trans and everything. And I don't know what is this phenomenon in Brazil that does this. I know some *travesti*s, even here in Bahia that when they are fifty, sixty, seventy years old, they start to become male again. Keeping their hair short.
>
> (Interviewee 2, February 27, 2012)

These are important issues, emphasising the effects of transphobia and the struggle to survive, crucially, the change in identity to be able to find employment. The masculinisation of *travesti*s and transwomen was also observed in other studies (Antunes & Mercadante, 2011):

> Old age is not valued, including among *travesti*s. It is as if the *travesti* lost her function when she gets old. So, they end up disappearing. Some say that there are some who grow old and start dressing like men again. They undergo a kind of 'de-transformation'. Others end up taking on other jobs, such as dressmakers, make-up artists, *bombadeiras* ((pumpers) people who apply industrial silicone among others), cooks,

> hairdressers, manicurists, *domésticas* (housekeepers), pimps, landlords, agents, artists, etc.
>
> (Antunes & Mercadante, 2011, p. 122, italics in the original)

The roles that older *travestis* play is another significant dimension, acting as counsellors, mothers, and godmothers, due to their knowledge of body techniques, as well as their life experience. As Antunes and Mercadante also observe (2011, pp. 116–117), 'their task is to initiate, protect and teach the younger ones to live as *travestis*'.

For both public policy and research, it is vital that we consider the issues highlighted in the interviews regarding ageing. The low life expectancy of *travestis* due to violence and social exclusion was a key factor observed in the research. Ageing was highlighted as having a direct impact on possibilities for employment (considering social), and the need to adapt, sometimes in bodily terms, through masculinisation. Prejudice experienced due to being elderly was also observed, while in other contexts, older *travestis* came to occupy a social position of 'godmother'. Finally, the effects of bodily transformation are often intensified in the elderly, and medical monitoring was seen as an important dimension. However, the transphobic environment, also present in some health care practice, was viewed as an obstacle when accessing health services. Various forms of marginalisation of the trans population were noted, from restrictions on their presence in public spaces to difficulties in accessing health services. Older *travestis* in this context are even more marginalised, 'they become old marginals', as interviewee 1 has observed.

4.3 Revisiting history: military dictatorship, AIDS and immigration

> The ideological construction of gender maintains male domination. If, in the context of colonial production, the subaltern subject has no history and cannot speak, the female subaltern subject is even more deeply in obscurity.
>
> (Spivak, 1988/2011, pp. 66–67)

Extending Spivak's (1988/2011) reflections and including the effects of cisgenderism (Ansara & Hegarty, 2011), we ask how the *travesti* and her experience are continuously marginalised and silenced, and crucially, what the possibilities are for her speaking and being heard without mediation. Taking these issues into account, I highlight the lived experience of *travestis* as they themselves tell it. While on one hand, their life stories over time are revealed, on the other, they testify to their marginalised position in society. This practice counteracts the production of a totalised history (Foucault, 1969/2002) by uncovering dimensions that are often excluded or overlooked, showing how subaltern groups are configured within totalising history as continuously marginalised, only being present on the periphery, and frequently pathologised or criminalised. Two aspects are emphasised in this sub-section: the history of transphobia and homophobia in Brazil since the 1960s and trans immigration in this context.

The excerpts below present several aspects involving the effects of institutional transphobia in the daily lives of *travestis*. The interviewees spoke of their cultural and social gatherings in a context of social exclusion, and the police and military violence during the military dictatorship in Brazil (1964–1985). One interviewee starts with the case of the *Turma OK*, an LGBT social club founded in 1961 that organised diverse initiatives such as meetings, parties and drag shows (Soliva, 2019).

> Formerly here in Rio de Janeiro, the history of *travestility*, started here with Key Francis, exactly, we founded the Key Francis human rights award. The Key Francis. *Turma Ok*[8] started with a group of five guys, that started Alberto, Adagoberto [Agildo Guimarães, Anuar Farah, José Rodrigues] started to get together before they became the *Turma Ok*. They started to get together, and they were persecuted by the police. They weren't *travestis*, they were homosexuals. It was the first house in Latin America, . . . the most important . . . Gay house. . . . It was inaugurated in 1966. Who did presentations in the house? Key Francis who was a transsexual, Eloá who died recently at eighty-six years of age, she was *travesti*, . . . Raquel Barbosa will turn eighty-one, Eloá will be eighty-five. We should honour this because this is a legend. When they say that, myth, that a *travesti* doesn't age, a *travesti* does. Eloá died three years ago at eighty-five. We have Raquel Barbosa who will be eighty-one. (Interviewee n. 3, July 23, 2011).
>
> [Key Francis] She was the first *travesti* in the *Turma OK* to start doing shows. . . . What happened? It was the army, it was the time of the dictatorship. Me, I am from a generation that came later, in 69. . . . But they suffered a lot. Why was that? They came in dressed as men, boys, young men and left dressed as women. The only one that really came out, who came out as she was, at that time was Rogéria,[9] this Angela Negliri and Cláudia Celeste.[10] Who weren't afraid. . . . And another, for the standard of that time, they really seemed to be the stereotypes the phenotype of women. . . . And Cláudia Celeste, wow, anyone who looked at Cláudia Celeste, she was a woman. The extravagant Rogéria with her hair was a great *travesti (travestisona)*, but she was of the feminine phenotype, because she already had breasts, she already had the stereotypes of a woman, because she took a lot of hormones, which at the time, we took Lindiol, we took Gestadinona, which was injectable and every doctor or pharmacist that administered it on a *travesti* at the time was stripped of their license or else they were arrested, they were arrested. At that time, I want to stress it clearly, at

that time, people thought that the military police, the institution of the military police has only existed for thirty years. We were commanded by the army. Those who arrested us were the army. Then the Military Police was established, the institution of the military police. . . . But who commanded was the army. So, simply for being gay, being gay, they already thought it was an affront. Now if you were a *travesti* of a woman, it was even more of an affront. But what happened? The *travesti* always had, there is a gaze from civil society, mainly regarding the relationship with men. (Interviewee 3, July 23, 2011).

What we have observed is at that time when the prostitutes needed to do this. So much so that there was that *marchinha* (Carnival song) "*De dia é Maria, de noite é João*" (By day it's Mary, by night it's John). This comparison was to modify this thing, because it was a conjuncture. People weren't used to seeing it. (Interviewee 2, personal interview, February 27, 2012).

They have to understand that if today they are in the street wearing skirts, they have to thank those who came before who were beaten with truncheons, went to prison, were shocked and hung from the *pau de arara* (a torture technique). I experienced all of this; we couldn't see a police car in the street. If we saw a police car on the street, one shouted to the other: Mona, look at the *'alibã'* [Yorubá language], then there was nobody left on the street. (Interviewee 1, February 8, 2012).

As I explained to you previously on the Yoruba language, that was how we defended ourselves against the police.

(Interviewee 3)

Here several important aspects stand out. Both police and routine day-to-day violence are clearly present. In this context, *Yorubá*, an African language, was employed as a form of communication to try to evade police violence. *Pajubá* or *Bajubá* is a form of language used and developed by the travestis, LGBT+ communities and other social groups, and it combines mostly Iorubá-Nagô, and French and English. Moreover, interviewees recall how in this setting, they 'performed' according to the situation they found themselves in, entering places 'dressed as men and leaving dressed as women'. The following fragment reveals certain dynamics associated with institutional transphobia and experiences on the street.

From the police, from the kids in the street, from the 'daddy's boys' (*filhinhos de papai*). The same violence that exists today existed in my time. We were arrested for loitering, for being in the streets without our ID.

Interviewer: And many of them didn't have ID?

The majority of those who were in the streets didn't have documents (ID), because *travestis* are always moving from one place to another,

> sometimes they are robbed, or they travel and lose their documents along the way. This always happens, sometimes you are on the street and a motorcyclist steals your bag, then you have to get a birth certificate in another state, and all this is expensive. Getting documents is very difficult for a *travesti.*
>
> (Interviewee 1, February 8, 2012)

The context of structural transphobia and the dynamics arising from it are notable in this extract. The interviewee highlighted several forms of ongoing violence, including institutional and day-to-day violence. These issues become visible in the form of the social vulnerability resulting from simply occupying urban spaces (police arrest and street violence) and the loss of their ID in this context.

Immigration, schooling and transphobia

> Travesti is always migrating from one place to another.
>
> (Interview 1, February 8, 2012)

Transphobia is a fundamental dimension of the experience of *travestis* in Brazil, which is part of the context in which immigration emerges as a possibility for survival and social mobility. Immigration refers to domestic migration, leaving their home town, while international migration, moving to other countries, involves preferably moving to destinations that especially guarantee greater security and possibility for social advancement. Experiences of transphobia during adolescence are also notable, with frequent dropping out of school, as well as often having to leave home and leave their hometown, also compounding the difficulty of these domestic and international migrations (Mountian, 2014a). In the extracts below, childhood and adolescent transphobia is highlighted:

> I thought I was a woman, until I went to school, and I saw that I wasn't a woman. Then I was ashamed to walk with my male friends and they would see that I wasn't a woman . . . I didn't go to the bathroom for fear that they would find out. (at the age of 7). (Interviewee 4, October 8, 2010).
>
> In my adolescence, today they say there is bullying, but there has been bullying for many years. I always had big buttocks and I suffered from this experience of bullying, . . . the boys waited till the end of the class to call me *bundudo* (big buttocks) and ran after me shouting . . . I wore a blouse covering [my back] because I was ashamed, afraid of the aggressions. I would cover my body for fear of these aggressions, the boys ran after me, there were many running after me. (Interviewee 4, October 8, 2010).

> When I left home I couldn't study any longer because it wasn't possible to reconcile my survival with study and work.
>
> (K., *travesti*) (Mountian, 2014a)

These experiences associated with transphobic violence suffered during childhood and adolescence at school are present in the experience of many *travestis*. Dropping out of school and expulsion from the family and the community were related by the interviewees as events that had a profound impact on their social vulnerability, as seen in another research (Mountian, 2014a).

Another crucial issue that was emphasised refers to the impact of AIDS on the trans community, from the sheer number of cases to the increased stigmatisation of LGBTQI+ people. The importance of LGBTQI+ activism for HIV prevention campaigns and interventions was highlighted, as also observed in the next section looking at the context of immigration.

> I started, like all of us, to use condoms in 1985 in Paris. Why was that? Because in our milieu, when AIDS began to infect *travestis*, it was an avalanche, they died, 2 or 3 per week. And it began . . . there was a big hotel called ABC where *travestis* settled in the ABC, many of the *travestis* who had flats began to sell their things, to sell furniture, their flats . . . they began to send money to Brazil . . . I saw *travestis* with atrophies, *travestis* without teeth. (Interviewee 3).
>
> There were no NGOs, there was no non-governmental organization, I was the pioneer there . . . I was responsible for all the *travestis*. . . and an avalanche of murdered *travestis* began . . . dying . . . (. . .) there was no more joy in the eyes of *travestis* . . . because it was death, they only talked about death and that *le sida* [in French], which was AIDS. So the nightclub was no longer full, I began to enter into a depressive state, that jungle of Bologna . . . an infectious jungle . . . it's like the Tijuca forest here . . . you enter the jungle with a cord, string so that you don't get lost . . . and the *travestis* buried their money, often when they were expelled . . . so to find where the money was they had to use a cord or mark it on a tree. So it was a stage in my life when I won a human rights prize from the Ministry of Health. What did I do? I began to distribute condoms, the *travestis* who were very sick began to live there in the shelter, I began to take the travestis to the shelter, where they were fed, bathed and could not go to the street to prostitute themselves, because if they went to the street to prostitute themselves they would put them on a plane and send them here to Brazil, that's what happened unfortunately with many who did not listen to me (Interviewee 3).
>
> So I made a decision, it was in 1989, I left France and went to live in Madrid, but I want to say that before I left Paris the French government gave me a human rights prize, I won this human rights prize . . . I was responsible, I distributed condoms, but my mental state couldn't handle it any more, all the glamour, everything I wanted to see I had

> already seen, and I went to live in Madrid. And I was also devastated (*assolada*) . . . all of Europe was devastated by AIDS, all Europe was devastated. I got tired, I started to do shows in Madrid, I won prizes in Madrid, I did shows in various places, I met the main people . . . the same life, but then I made up my mind, in 1992 I left Europe. I left, I made a decision and left. I went to São Paulo, where I was born.
>
> (Interviewee 3)

Studies on *travestis* and transgender people and immigration are still scarce (Carrijo, 2011; Teixeira, 2011; Vartabedian, 2014a). Vartabedian (2014b) emphasises the notion of 'trans immigration' to define the phenomenon of migratory processes that deal with the specificities of the experience of trans people (*travestis*, transsexuals, transgenders and others). For the analysis of trans immigration, it is essential to take into account the transphobic character of their place of origin, of the destination and throughout the trajectory, considering the impact of the dynamics of race, social class and age. Limitations on employment for trans people and violence at diverse levels has been a great concern, with immigration being seen as a possibility for escaping violence and finding means for survival (Pereira, 2021). Immigration is sought in the promise of freedom and respect for their sexual identities, and as a possibility of employment and economic growth (Vartabedian, 2014b). The possibility of living less transphobic lives is highlighted in other studies. Furthermore, Pelúcio (2011) shows that there is an understanding that European men are more likely to publicly 'assume' (*assumiram*) a relationship with a trans person than in Brazil.

> Thus, besides being able to find a 'real man', Europe could create a possibility to leave prostitution and provide a life within a script that they classify as 'normal' – raise a family, move around during the day without experiencing embarrassment and be worthy of the same kindnesses that men dedicate to biological women.
>
> (Pelúcio, 2011, p. 187)

Moreover, immigration can be seen as a doorway to a 'promised land' where other experiences can be found. Pelúcio (2011, p. 186) argues that they are also 'seeking wider horizons for cosmopolitan experiences that can be translated into contact with different cultures, language learning, various cultural codes, in addition to the possibility of enjoying places, tours, food, pleasures and people'. The possibility of experiencing other forms of relationships with personal security and labour inclusion was highlighted as an important aspect for national and international immigration, as seen in the following:

> The dream of every *travesti* was to go to Europe, all of them. I had many friends who went, I had many friends who died there, who came back infected and died here. (Interviewee 1, February 8, 2012)

> Nowadays you see it here in Salvador. Most of the *travestis* that are here in Salvador go to São Paulo, go to Rio [de Janeiro], go to Belo Horizonte. And today there is not only a migration from these cities here, from the countryside there always has been. So, if you arrive today in a capital . . . there is less of this here now, but if you arrive in Recife today and ask, the majority of those *travestis* in Recife who work, they came from small towns. They come from small towns in the interior of the country and come to Recife. In Salvador we also find this, but not as often as in other states. What they're doing now, as Europe is in crisis now, they're jumping from state to state. They go from Salvador to Belo Horizonte, from Belo Horizonte to Curitiba, from Curitiba to Florianópolis. They keep migrating, within Brazil itself. But on their own means. There may be some that even travel if someone helps them financially. This thing of national trafficking. But the majority of them that I know, they pay their own way. They get money, buy a ticket, call someone who has a house there, one of those houses (*pensões*) that are around. Then they end up settling and go to work there for a while.
>
> (Interviewee 2, February 27, 2012)

In these extracts, various forms of migration experienced by *travestis* are observed, both national and international, particularly from rural towns to capital cities. Considering the various forms of transphobic violence, immigration provides the promise of social ascension and security, highlighting the issue of the intrinsic relationship between politics of sexuality and immigration. In this context, we once again note how the intersections of gender, sexuality, race, social class and age become fundamental for an analysis that seeks to comprehend diverse experiences of immigration and access to services.

Present times

In the interviews conducted, many interviewees highlighted important changes in the social condition of *travestis* today. Difficulties stemming from transphobia remain paramount in the experience of trans people, *travestis*, transwomen and transmen; however, interviewees also emphasised some advances in terms of citizenship and human rights compared to earlier years.

> Things are becoming clearer, people are respecting each other more, the police are respecting us more, but the evangelical people are not. (Interviewee 5, February 27, 2012)
>
> In the past we almost didn't go out during the day, it was much more difficult. Nowadays, things have become a little bit easier for them. I see girls on the bus, travelling and walking in the mall even though they are criticised and humiliated, because I see people looking, poking and laughing.
>
> (Interviewee 1, February 8, 2012)

In these responses, the advances in human rights are notable, where despite the continuation of a transphobic environment, some *travestis* and transwomen have begun to experience greater social integration with somewhat greater ease than during prior historical periods. However, according to the interviewees, while some sectors of society have begun to respect *travestis*, there is continued prejudice felt from parts of the evangelical community, underlining how religious intolerance impacts into transphobia.

It is important to be aware of the effects of transphobia and its dynamics in public spaces, particularly the (non) presence of *travestis* in public during daytime hours. In this sense, one can reflect on how public space is gendered, when seen within the framework of the invisibility of *travestis* and transgender populations in public spaces, a social constraint that extends to accessing formal employment, education, health services and security (Mountian, 2014c). Given this, it becomes relevant to question when *travestis* become visible, when their presence is pathologised and criminalised and when their absence is normalised (Phoenix, 1987).

In relation to health services, it is worth pointing out that trans people are often visible in spaces associated with 'transsexualising' (gender affirmative) processes, and in specific areas of health often related to sexual health. As Amaral et al. (2014, p. 304) observe, attention has focused on preventive health initiatives, mostly perceived as directly related to AIDS by professionals and governments, and assistance associated with drug use and crime prevention.

It is important to consider, therefore, the dynamics of visibility experienced by *travestis*, transwomen and transmen, interrogating the normalised absence that all too often characterises this experience and the forms of exclusion to which this population is subjected. Such an analysis is crucial for combating transphobia and for avoiding the reproduction of this marginalised social position in the provision of health services and in everyday relations.

Final considerations

The issues raised by the elderly *travestis* who participated in our research included several aspects such as ageing, body, immigration, labour market, health, education, history and transphobia. All these aspects open up numerous questions, being essential therefore to consider the specific social contexts and their power relations in the analysis. In this case, understanding the specificities of transphobic social contexts and its effects on the possibilities for trans ageing becomes paramount.

The stories that we heard from older *travestis* were marked by violence and prejudice even in the most banal and everyday situations. This also often involved institutional or state violence, which also revealed the power dynamics under coercive external conditions. Social exclusion was noticeable in the marginalisation, ostracism and silence, produced within specific dynamics of visibility and invisibility in public spaces, an issue which also has to be further analysed for transmen and trans masculinities.

Their interaction with health services was characterised by an experience of difficulties stemming from transphobia, with a focus on sexually transmitted disease, and a failure to account for the specificities of trans people and their bodies that undergo specific changes, an issue that is particularly important for ageing trans people and those with disabilities. The way that health service providers, particularly psy professionals, engage with trans people has to be carefully considered, as specific moral biases may continue to be present, which can reproduce excluding discursive positions. The encounter with the trans population elucidates the situated therapeutic culture, in which the trans specificities are often not considered.

Transphobia must be taken as a fundamental issue in the relationship of *travestis* with ageing, from what it is to be considered elderly (over 40 years old), to the need of health services that are not transphobic. The specificities of older trans people have to be taken into account, including bodily changes stemming from ageing and the relationship with prostheses, plastics surgeries, hormones and silicone that also affect their own relationship with their body, due to the effects on health and the need for 'touch-ups' (Siqueira, 2004). It is therefore fundamental to guarantee access to health services free of transphobia, as well as services that have a specific understanding of the effects of bodily interventions. This highlights the continued need to obtain more robust and detailed statistical data about ageing and life expectancy in this community.

In light of the institutional transphobia which limits or bars access to education, work and health for this population, sex work arises as a social space 'allowed' to *travestis*, as well as some professions stereotypically associated with them (such as hairdresser, manicurist, etc.). In sex work, according to the interviewees, there is a certain age limit, leading to a situation of greater financial vulnerability for older *travestis*. Consequently, the issue of how some *travestis* masculinise themselves to be able to work also arose, as an aspect that generates significant questions surrounding the possibilities for the identities of older *travestis*. Moreover, it would be relevant to research the impact of retirement on the health (Mountian & Diaz, 2020) of the trans population.

Regarding their personal testimony, it is important to locate the body of the *travesti* in a historical context. In the interviews undertaken, most *travestis* were found to have moved to a new city or country, and according to their accounts, this migration was directly related to local homophobia and transphobia. Immigration was often understood by the *travesti* population as a search for less transphobic environments, seeking greater social mobility and security. In this sense, it was notable how the *travesti* body is a sexually marked one, conferring a specific discursive space (a non-place, or one with little room, a closet) (on the politics of the closet, see Sedgwick, 1991); somehow, the non-space is continuously re-enacted through ongoing transphobic social reactions to which *travestis* are subjected. As a counterpart, in the interviews, resistance and struggle against prejudice and discrimination were strongly emphasised. In this sense, the trans body also informs the debate surrounding the possibility of widening and resisting power relations based on binary gender divisions. Trans performativity should be understood through the intersections of social categories of gender, sexuality, race, class, disability and age. As such, the way in which the effects of transphobia are inseparable from those of racism, classism, ableism and ageism becomes evident. Experiences were reported from various parts of Brazil, with specific regional dynamics; however, in all interviews, the testimony was marked by confrontation and resistance to various forms of local violence, including religious intolerance.

The issue that we are dealing with here is in a double sense a 'marginal' one, not only in relation to the social position occupied by *travesti*s but also in the academic area, such as in Psychology. There also a duplicity can be observed, not only in terms of the access of travestis to the university but also in relation to research about transwomen and men.

It is important, therefore, to give voice to these groups and highlight how transphobic and homophobic relations produce subjectivity, seen in the reproduction of these relations as well as in the forms of resistance to LGBTQIAphobic discourses, allowing us to reflect on discursive shifts in hierarchical gender relations.

It is necessary, therefore, to develop research and implement public policy in this area, which would take into account the specific demands, dynamics, intersectional dimensions and local contexts pertinent to the *travesti* and trans community; and to include trans people, *travestis*, transsexual and transgender women, transsexual and transgender men and trans masculine people as active subjects in academic research, in the development of public policy and in historiography.

Notes

1 It is important to note that these numbers are from before 2018.
2 This chapter is based on the article Mountian, I. (2015a). 'Aspectos sobre travestilidade e envelhecimento: história, corpo e imigração'. *Quaderns de Psicologia*, Vol. 17, No 3, 31–44.
3 To maintain their anonymity the interviews will be referred to using numbering.
4 I will utilise the definition of Keila Simpson (2021) for *Travesti*. 'Não existe definição na minha modesta opinião (até rimou). Sigamos que para mim, ser e se identificar como *Travesti* além de reforçar uma identidade política é um estado de espírito que convive comigo desde que me entendo por gente, obviamente que nesse debate há muitas complexidades e considero a maioria delas, mas essa de termo X atrelado a termo Y não passa de apagamento. Vamos dar nome às coisas'.
5 Translated by the author.
6 Translated by the author.
7 Translated by the author.
8 https://www.youtube.com/watch?v=xGLIEItYhRY https://www.youtube.com/watch?v=JjOUZ4g6yTg
https://www.uol.com.br/universa/reportagens-especiais/respeite-as-bichas-talkei/#page2 https://www.tropicuir.org/turma-ok/
9 Known actress and TV presenter (Soliva, 2018)
10 First *travesti* to participate in soap opera, actress, dancer. https://en.identidadesmarginais.com/claudia-celeste
https://revistageni.org/06/diva-que-incomoda-claudia-celeste/

5 Discourses on drug addiction and gender

In this chapter, we will further explore the imaginary of women and drugs, primarily based on the results of the research undertaken for my doctoral thesis. The interviews highlighted a number of key issues surrounding the role of gender in drug use and treatment contexts, while the position of the researcher during fieldwork undertaken in a medical institution was also explored, concerning the participant's response to the researcher who is a psychologist (see more in Mountian, 2017a). The interviews were conducted at in-patient clinics (private and public) and in informal settings.

The history of medicine and psychiatry shows the situatedness of mental health classifications and the production of a therapeutic culture. The notion of drug addiction seen in Chapter 2 underlined the historical construction of drug addiction and highlighted moral values imbued in them, in that the notion of addiction has come to signify any kind of repetitive and compulsive behaviour. This mental illness diagnosis carries with it a stigma which contributes to constructing the subject's identity, that is as drug user or ex-drug user. Therefore, a critical reading of how drug addiction has been conceived and utilised becomes crucial. As discussed earlier, while there must be a clear awareness of the potential individual suffering of those involved in drug use circles, we also argue that the effects resulting from specific conceptions of addiction on the subject's experience and on research and treatment in this area must also be interrogated.

Through a critical discursive analysis, the relations between gender, sexuality, class, race and age within the notion of drug addiction will be further investigated, underlining the limited/limiting views on male drug users, the over stigmatisation of women and LGBTQI+ people, and how drug treatment and research often ignore these social categories within specific contexts. The effects of LGBTQIphobia in drug services will also be considered as well as the impact of moral conceptions on women, which stigmatise and act as a barrier for women and LGBTQI+ people when seeking help.

DOI: 10.4324/9780429263415-8

5.1 Social imaginary of the drug addict

Discourses surrounding drug use are often morally saturated, oscillating between good and evil, which can affect research and treatment and crucially, the social imaginary related to drug users. In this manner, binary discursive positions of victim and enemy are frequently in play when considering this phenomenon. As such, it becomes relevant to question how and when these imaginary positions are evoked. Medical discourses, for example, position the drug user as a victim of the disease of addiction, and thus as being in need of medical care. This contrasts with other approaches that understand the drug user as the enemy, for example, due to potentially harming others. From this perspective, this may involve their inclusion in criminal legislation or in religious discourses as immoral individuals. The reproduction of these binary oppositions can be seen in common-sense notions that circulate through the signifiers 'mad, bad, or sad'. These viewpoints situate the subject in discursive positions, under a specific gaze, producing subjective outcomes. Here, we will be focusing on the signifier 'drug user', considering its stigmatising effect, as well as investigating when it is used as a mental health classification and identity.

Stigma derives from *stigmata*, referring to a mark on the body, which irrevocably identifies the person with some disgrace that has befallen them. For the ancient Greeks, it would be inflicted as a punishment for treason, or escaping from a master, marking the person rather than the deed as spoiled. Warner (1999) claims that this would be equivalent to Goffman's modern metaphor for 'spoiled identity'. This idea of 'spoiled identity' could also be seen here as evoking the dispute between medical and religious models of drug addiction.

It is relevant to question how this 'spoiled identity' operates in relation to the self-identification of drug users as addict, drug user or ex-user. We ask when this naming is used as the only identity of the subject, limiting their discursive possibilities, since the subject identification is reduced to only the relationship with the drug, circulating around this specific signifier and not allowing other forms of identification, that is, when one is a user, one is always a user or becomes an ex-*user*, as is often the case in medical and religious therapeutic centres. This perspective contrasts to other understandings of drug use (Mountian, 2005), such as the sociological view on social rituals (Zinberg, 1984; South, 1999; Gusfield, 1987), and through the notion of habitus (Bourdieu, 1977; Sedgwick, 1992); and psychoanalytic conceptualisations that aim to increase the space for understandings of drug use and drug users, such fetishism (Freud, 1977; Lacan, 1995), repetition (Olievenstein, 1989; Lacan, 1994), *jouissance* and transgression (Lacan, 1992) and the relationship to the drug object (Olievenstein, 1989; Gurfinkel, 1996).

The notion of the scapegoat, associated with that of stigma, is also relevant in this context. It is a widely used concept in group therapy models, interpreted as emotional displacement, a defence mechanism and as a group indication of projective identification (Scheidlinger, 1982; Taylor & Rey, 1953).

The term scapegoat from the Hebrew 'goat for Azazel' refers to the Day of Atonement when one or two chosen goats were symbolically loaded with the sins of the Jewish people, with one goat being pushed off a cliff, and the other sacrificed to the Lord (Scheidlinger, 1982). In Ancient Greece, the scapegoat was part of religious practice to protect communities from plagues, famine and other threats. Sacrificing humans for these purposes, scapegoats were selected and then sacrificed. Significantly, the person who was sacrificed as a scapegoat was called *pharmakos* (Szasz, 1975), representing the expulsion of evil from the body and from the city (Derrida, 1997).

This notion of scapegoat (and *pharmakos*) is relevant to understand the current imaginary associated with drugs and the moral grounds for the 'war on drugs' in relation to the moral conflict between good and evil that the *pharmakos* embodies, good when it is related to cure, being venerated and surrounded by care, and evil when it embodies qualities of being venomous and causing fear (Derrida, 1997).

The dynamics of scapegoating and stigmatisation has been debate by a number of authors. Xiberras (1989) discusses this double movement, that is, society labels drug users as scapegoats and they accept it, as hard intoxication is seen here as the prototype of non-adaptation. Xiberras also observes that the stigmatisation of drug users can lead them to intensify practices of intoxication. Similarly, Dally (1996) points out that addicts (whether patients or not) have low self-esteem, which is also related to the way they are viewed in society and by medical institutions. 'They still feel they have to play the part of the degraded, dying creatures that society wants them to be' (p. 201). This process has effects for the subject and drug prevention and treatment measures, for example, in terms of difficulties in forming pressure groups, even for providing information about drugs, as it is regarded as an immoral act.

In these discourses, the social context of the drug user is obliterated, positioning them as a pathological subject. This dynamic displaces the problematic of the social context onto the drug use itself, whereby structural power relations remain unchallenged. Social relations that are mediated by distinctions of class, race and gender have, therefore, to be adequately considered. Furthermore, it is important to consider the differences between consuming and producing countries regarding drug policy and criminal approaches.

As already observed, the social imaginary surrounding the drug user is constantly informed by the discursive binary of either victim or enemy. As such, the subject would be either a *victim* of bad influences, neurological dysfunctions and the drug habit itself, or an *enemy* who is prejudicial to others due to drug-related crimes or by harming the health of others, participating in the illegal drug trade (consuming or dealing).

The conception of drug taking as immoral, already discussed in Chapter 2, was noticeable in still prevalent discourses surrounding drugs as a sin, disease and later as criminal. Shapiro (1999) argues that the use of drugs such as solvents and heroin are regarded as marginal activities associated with 'urban deprivation and social dislocation' (p. 18). Although other forms of drug use have challenged this image, such as the use of ecstasy by youth, the stereotypical conception of the drug user continues to be that of 'mad, bad or sad' (ISDD, 1976)" (1999), or as Young (1971) observes, drug users are regarded as immoral, lacking norms or as sick.

The signifiers 'mad, bad and sad' in the field of drug addiction shift between discourses and operate strategically depending on the context. These categories illustrate key discourses surrounding drugs and drug users that are deeply entrenched in medical, legal and religious discourses. Crucially, these signifiers and discourses should not be taken as the only available ones, or understood in isolation, as they often appear in tandem.

When deconstructing the 'mad, bad and sad' trope, it is possible to locate the signifier mad within medical discourse, constituting the image of the 'victim' of drug addiction; 'bad', as the 'enemy', associated with criminality, that is, with the legal sphere; and 'sad' when viewed through the lens of moral discourses evoked (i.e., religious morality), also used as 'bad'. These dynamics operate differently according to the intersections between gender, sexuality, race, class, disability and age distinctions. The interplay of these categories generates specific subjective effects, situating subjects within a limited field of possible identifications and affecting drug policy and drug treatment.

5.2 Social imaginary of women and drugs in Brazil

Hegemonic discourses on drugs based on religious/moral, medical and legal perspectives were seen in terms of primitivising (working class, immigrant), orientalising (upper class, immigrant) and sexualising (gender and sexuality) conceptions of drug use.

Here I focus on gender and drug use, from the discourse analysis of visual images and interviews undertaken for my PhD thesis (Mountian, 2005) and based on the book *Cultural Ecstasies: drugs, gender and social imaginary* (Mountian, 2013a). The main issues that will be explored here are: the effects of women traditionally seen as the primary victims of drug or as perpetuating drug use. The dynamics of invisibility and visibility of women and drugs regarding the sexualised gaze directed at women, (re)producing the discursive positions of the 'mother' and the 'fallen woman'. And finally, how, paradoxically, drug use was seen in some contexts as a site for female empowerment. Specific aspects concerning LGBTQIA+ people will be highlighted, particularly in terms of the effects of LGBTQIAphobia in this field. This analysis will outline elements for drug policy and therapeutic interventions.

A Foucauldian analysis is undertaken (Parker, 1997; Foucault, 1991), drawing on feminist and post/decolonial research. The images are seen not only as a product of the social context, but also as productive (Rose, 2001). The notion of social imaginary employed here derives from Lacan's (1991) imaginary dimension and Castoriadis' (1991) notion of social imaginary (signification). The focus on the social imaginary, in this case of drug users and gender, enables an approach in which images, fantasies, (mis)recognition and illusions are taken as relevant to the constitution of subjectivity. These elements both constitute and are constituted by society.

'Drugs', 'addiction' and 'drug users' are read as shifting signifiers, and there are no definitive structures or stopping points, but rather chains of association or deferred meaning (Silva, 2000). In these terms, these signifiers are not approached from an essentialist framework but rather viewed as socially constructed (Macey, 1994).

The object 'drug' will be seen here as a conflicting signifier, an object structured according to power relations, producing specific 'bodies of discourse' (i.e. medical, legal, religious). In the same vein, as seen in Chapter 1, gender is understood as performative, as an acquired process and not as a situated fixed biological concept (Butler, 1993). In this sense, the emergence of gender is an outcome of this process of social construction understood within the intersection of key categories of sexuality, class, race, age, disability and others. Therefore, I will focus on aspects concerning the social roles and expectations associated with women, and not on essentialist or prescriptive accounts. As Allen (1986, p. 104) points out,

> It is important to understand that these central problems (which are concerned, amongst other things, with issues of dependency, neediness, anger, the body, control and guilt) are not conceived simply as problems to which women are prone, but as problems to which they are prone as women.

The term drugs refers to any substance, legal or illegal, for recreational or medicinal use, that is exogenous substances that provokes a functional and/or structural effect in the body. Juxtaposing discourses on drugs with gender, a number of known gendered signifiers are repeated in this field, such as the Other, madness and dependency, leading to a feminisation of the drug user, and operating in specific ways with women. While these aspects will be further debated, however they are socially and culturally specific and concepts that should not be read as unique, a-historical, universal category, but rather as indicative perspectives, that vary according to the social context in which they are produced.

Women as the 'other': madness and dependency

Here I analyse how discourses on drug users as 'infantile', 'immature', 'weak'; 'dependent' and 'out of control' intersect with gender, characteristics typically seen as female. These aspects ('infantile', 'immature', 'weak', 'dependent', 'out of control') are often attributed to the subject position of the 'Other', a position commonly given to 'women' are commonly portrayed and constituted in social and psychological spaces (Burman, 2000; Nieves, 1994).

Reflecting on power in discourse and on the polarisations produced within the discursive dynamics surrounding women and drugs, I draw on some categories outlined by Burman (1999) in relation to three binary dimensions of the hierarchical relationship between children and adults: innocence vs. experience; dependency vs. autonomy; and spontaneity vs. reflectiveness. These antagonistic categories can be seen in the imaginary in relation to women, or to what are in some sense considered to be 'good', 'expected' or 'common' qualities in 'usual' feminine traits (i.e. innocence, dependency, spontaneity), characteristics that also appear in the intersections with discourses on drugs.

Discourses on drug use evoke ideas such as dependency, moral weakness and immaturity, which are opposed to self-control and reasoning. The drug user is seen as 'infantile', not able to postpone pleasure and dependent (as the classification of drug dependency itself). As Young (1971) highlights, 'the undersocialised drugtaker is seen in Freudian terms to have a weak superego, an inadequate ego – of a man – lack of proper masculine identification' (p. 53).

This conception of dependency becomes particularly problematic when it is overlaid with the question of gender, since traditionally, women are socialised into dependency, such that 'in the traditional discursive construction of heterosexuality, "man" is positioned as powerful, and "woman" as passive and beholden to man' (Ussher, 1998, p. 151). Control operates in contradictory ways, as Ettorre (1989) argues, although the social expectation for women is to behave in the traditional expected manner, that is, as dependent, yet there is 'an interesting incompatibility between the social expectation for women to be dependent and the need for all women to be "in control"' (p. 105). In this way, at the same time that there is this imaginary of uncontrollability and emotional spontaneity in relation to women, it is also expected that they should be in control, that is of their passions, desires and household.

In this sense, it is relevant to consider how discourses on 'madness' and women have been traditionally related, i.e. connected with sexual realms, with emotionality and vulnerability are traditionally being associated with women, as discussed in Chapter 2. Discourses on the female biology appear intertwined with the social roles attributed to women. As such, the characteristics of 'madness' are those found in the female experience, while it also reveals the position of the Other that women came to occupy. Moreover, women who do not correspond to the expected dependence and passive roles, and particularly those who transgress these social norms, may be viewed as having a mental illness. This dynamic has effects on the way that drug taking is viewed; crucially, this imaginary is socially specific, and how it varies across class and race is fundamental for the analysis, for example, how Black women, poor women and LBTQI+ people are seen regarding the 'female' 'fragility'.

Sexualised gaze and drug discourses

Female deviance is often associated with sexual deviance, which also reveals the social role reserved for women, and crucially, producing a specific gaze on women, invariably a sexualised one. Addiction in this way would be seen as a rejection of their sex-role stereotype, as women typically seen as bad mothers (contrasting with an idealised image of motherhood, Callaghan, 2015), or bad women (i.e. prostitutes, lesbians). As Campbell (2000, p. 154) highlights, 'Women's drug use is shown up in popular culture as a symptom of other feminised forms of female deviance, such as prostitution or lesbianism', that is as the feminised Other.

Hence deviance is commonly associated with sexual deviance, fitting within the more general polarised discursive binary of victim and enemy that discourses about drug users evoke. In the case of women, it is possible to highlight the particular sexualised version of this binary between the positions of the 'mother' and the 'fallen woman'. On the one hand, 'fallen woman' refers to those women who are regarded as hyper-sexual, 'not behaving as girls' or 'not behaving as proper girls', here implying terms such as 'tramp', 'lush' and 'whore', in line with the trope of 'rampant sexuality' figure (Finkelstein, 1996, p. 33). On the other hand, the discursive position of the 'bad mother' carries with it the view of women who are 'seen as potentially "sexless", uncaring for their children or as irresponsible wives, not considering the needs of their husbands' (Ettorre, 1989, p. 105). In these terms, the only drug use that is compatible with the stereotype of the 'proper lady' is the medicinal and/or cosmetic use of drugs, for example the use of tranquilisers and sliming pills, among others.

Psychoanalysis provides further insights when analysing these two images: of the 'mother' and 'fallen woman', psychoanalysis brings some further insights. Due to its marginal position in discourse, the feminine represents what is symbolised or not, what can be controlled, what can be subverted (Frosh, 1995). Moi (1985, p. 167) argues that within western culture women are neither inside or outside, neither known nor unknown, which gives rise to the creation of two basic discursive formations: women as the dark and chaotic (Lilith or the whore of Babylon), or as worthy of veneration due to being pure and close to nature (Virgins and Mothers of God). 'Whichever tendency dominates, "woman" here is a product of imagination, literally the imaginary; a fantasy that holds masculinity in place' (in Frosh, 1995, p. 293). This makes clear, therefore, the discursive position of the Other that 'women' occupy.

So far two aspects were emphasised: first, how the imaginary of the drug user is connected to that of the female (e.g. 'dependent', 'weak', 'mad', 'out of control'), and how the sexualised gaze operates in relation to women, seen as pure and venerated or as a fallen woman, imaginary positions that hold women in the discursive place of the Other.

> Feminist work has held up the dominant construction of the ideal mother (one in which women are constructed as selfless, nurturing, subsuming their own needs to attend to their children's) for scrutiny, arguing that it is often illusory, partial, and divisive.
>
> (Craig & O'Dell, 2011, p. 1)

It is worth considering the dynamics of the sexualised gaze of mother and fallen women for the development of research and public policy. In the interviews undertaken for the doctoral research (Mountian, 2005), for example, how these discourses operate in relation to emotions, in this case, of shyness and shame can be seen. This can be observed in the following extract:

> K.[1] (Why do women feel shame?) It is cultural, the woman, it is a problem of education, of upbringing etc., I believe that the next generations of girls as it is happening nowadays, that has so many problems with alcoholism, they drink together with the boys, get together a group of girls, they go out drinking in the bar and that's it. It is because they have another kind of mentality, another kind of education, it is another culture, it's something else (*negócio*). The older women no, they have more, they had an education. You know, where it was put this shame, really. Until only a little while ago, women didn't smoke in the street, *né*,[2] not to mention drinking. She drinks when she is with her husband, when she is with her boyfriend, but even then she doesn't exaggerate, because it is ugly (it's trashy, right?) (*fica feio* entendeu). It's a cultural matter really, a serious business (*negócio sério*). And for the woman who has an drinking problem, it's inside the house, until she finds help, you see that is a complicated problem (*negócio*), because for the man it's more obvious, but not for the woman, she is at home. Or the son runs away from home, somehow society hears about it, but never by herself, hardly ever by herself. So much so, that she reaches a point, the most serious point, that she starts to go out drinking, and falls over, then people get to know that woman has a story with alcohol.

There are important issues raised by K., highlighting the consequences of the (in)visibility of women in public, such that while they may be drinking alone at home, they only become 'visible' when the situation is 'out of control'. The way that shame operates for women is crucial for drug prevention and treatment, and outreach for older women. Moreover, the image of the older woman who drinks might be seen as incompatible with what is socially expected from them.

Women and nation

The social position of women in nation is typically related to the representation of social and moral norms, as the 'keepers' of society's morality, embodied in the traditional social roles of mothers and carers. Yuval-Davis (1997, p. 2) suggests that women 'reproduce nations, biologically, culturally and symbolically'. However, as although women are an essential part of the nation, they are excluded from the political arena, while the private sphere is considered politically irrelevant (McClintock, 1995); in many countries, women are kept outside institutional political power, having little presence in politics. In this sense, while women are located outside the public/political realms, they are seen as representatives of the reproduction of cultural morality, whereby they reproduce, maintain and symbolise the 'motherland' (Yuval-Davis, 1997).

The place of women as moral agents is also derived from the (feminised) body politic, 'to ensure a strong imperial race' (McDonald, 1994, p. 22). It is interesting to highlight the position of women as cultural reproducers of nation, especially for older women, who accorded this position, are expected to govern and adopt the appropriate behaviour. Therefore, according to this symbolic position, *drugs represent a special threat to nation, family and women themselves* (in the same way that homosexuality, prostitution and obscenity do (Warner, 1996)). That is, by using drugs, they threaten not only their own lives but also those of their families (especially children), and that of the nation, (re)producing or giving birth to an unruly and disorderly society.

It is relevant to note how in the U.K. and U.S. between the 1920s and 50s women were viewed as the main victims of drugs, while a connection between female drug use and moral degradation was highlighted, as seen in Chapter 2. This imaginary is also related to the fear of intermarriage (Kohn, 1992; Campbell, 2000), which represents another threat to the nation (reflecting among other issues a biological conception of nation). Littlewood and Lipsedge (1989, p. 42) point out that in the US until 1967, seventeen states had laws against intermarriage. 'A new technical language developed to control "miscegenation", utilizing such apparently precise terms as half-breed, hybrid, mulatto and octaroon'. Campbell (2000) underlines the fear of racial mixing in the U.S. at this time, with drug policies developed aiming to protect white women, and thereby intensifying the dangerousness attributed to black men. This is also due to the idea that white women were less resistant both to the pleasure and harm resulting from drugs. In this sense, one physician of that time went so far as to note that 'a delicate female having light blue eyes and flaxen hair, possesses, according to my observation the maximum susceptibility' (Kane *apud* Campbell, 2000, p. 68). Within femininity itself, therefore, gradations of susceptibility could be determined based on an apprehension of certain traits which *appear* to approximate the subject to an even greater degree towards that 'permeability' characteristic of women.

This particular social imaginary associated with women, which (re)produces the discursive position of female victimisation and moral degradation was portrayed in the media, literature and movies (see Mountian, 2013a, 2005). This can be seen in the analysis of the movies *Reefer Madness* (1934) and *Marihuana* (1936), part of the trend of US exploitation movies[3] from the 1930s, 40s and 50s, which draw on these particular imaginaries regarding drug use.

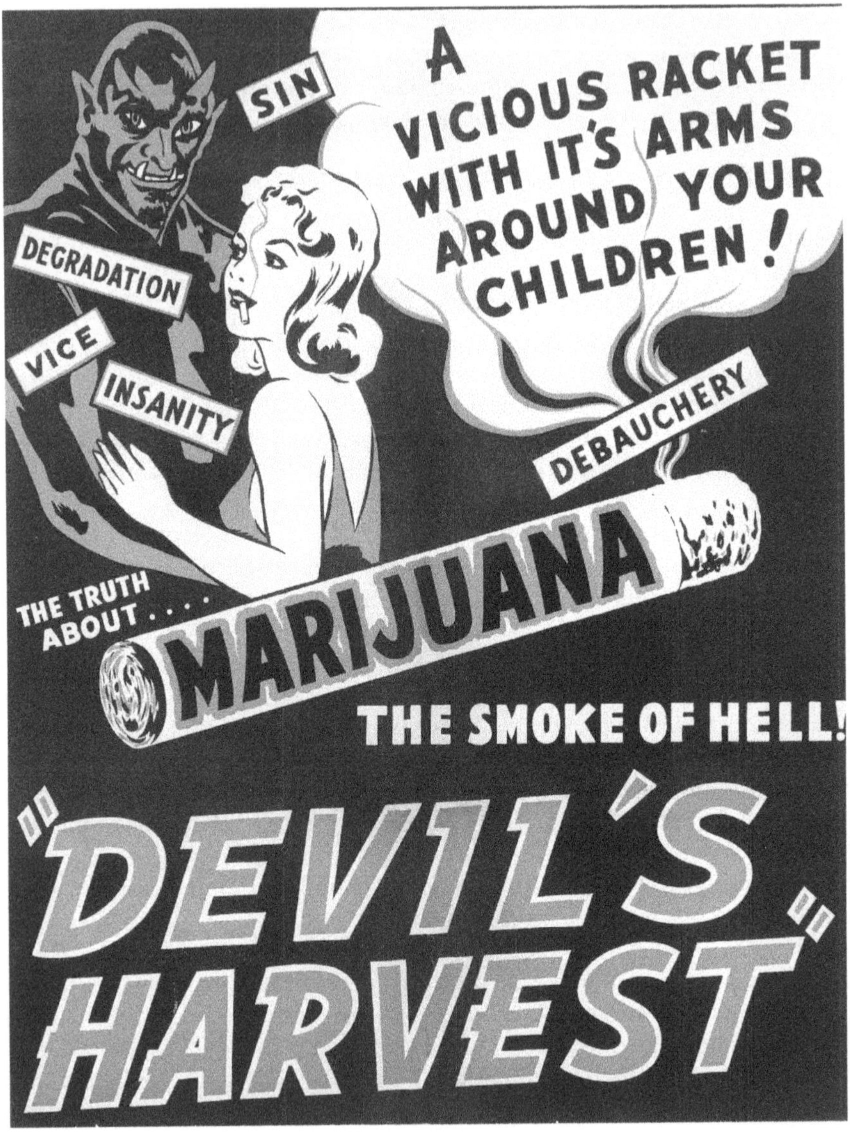
SIN
A VICIOUS RACKET WITH IT'S ARMS AROUND YOUR CHILDREN!
DEGRADATION
VICE
INSANITY
DEBAUCHERY
THE TRUTH ABOUT....
MARIJUANA
THE SMOKE OF HELL!
"DEVIL'S HARVEST"

Figure 5.1 Marihuana (1934)

Notes: The images in this sub-section were retrieved from www.imagesjournal.com/issue08/features/exploitation/in May/2003

'Degradation', 'vice', 'sin' and 'debauchery' are the tropes that make up the highly stigmatised context, where women are portrayed as either entrapped and victimised or as a threat evoking the idea of 'bad' or 'fallen women' (also suggested by their attire). Furthermore, within this image it is possible to interrogate a sort of racialised discourse involving the image of the devil, evoking the idea of fear of intermarriage. It is also relevant to note the text: Marijuana – 'A vicious racket with its arms around your children', which depicts a blonde woman, evoking the imaginary of women as infantile and dependent, being close to children (also cultivating the imaginary of drug users as dependent and infantile).

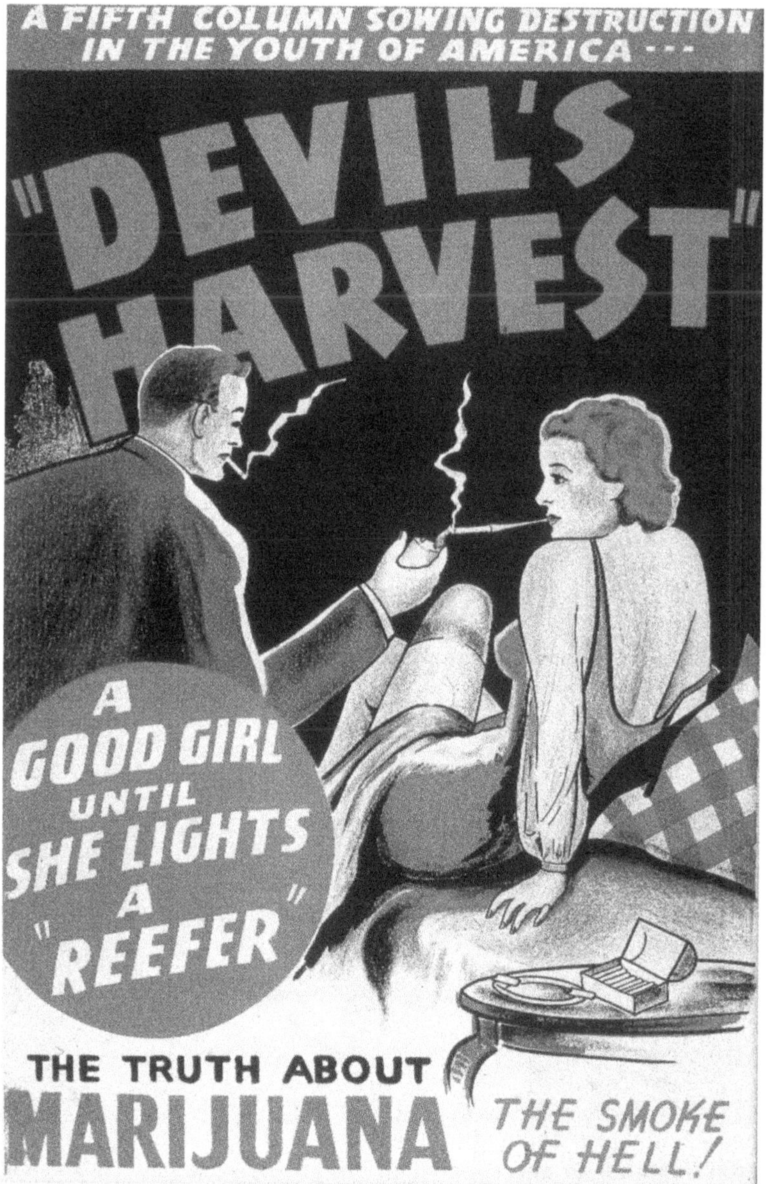
A FIFTH COLUMN SOWING DESTRUCTION
IN THE YOUTH OF AMERICA ---
"DEVIL'S HARVEST"
A GOOD GIRL UNTIL SHE LIGHTS A "REEFER"
THE TRUTH ABOUT
MARIJUANA
THE SMOKE OF HELL!

Figures 5.2a and 5.2b *Marihuana* (1934)

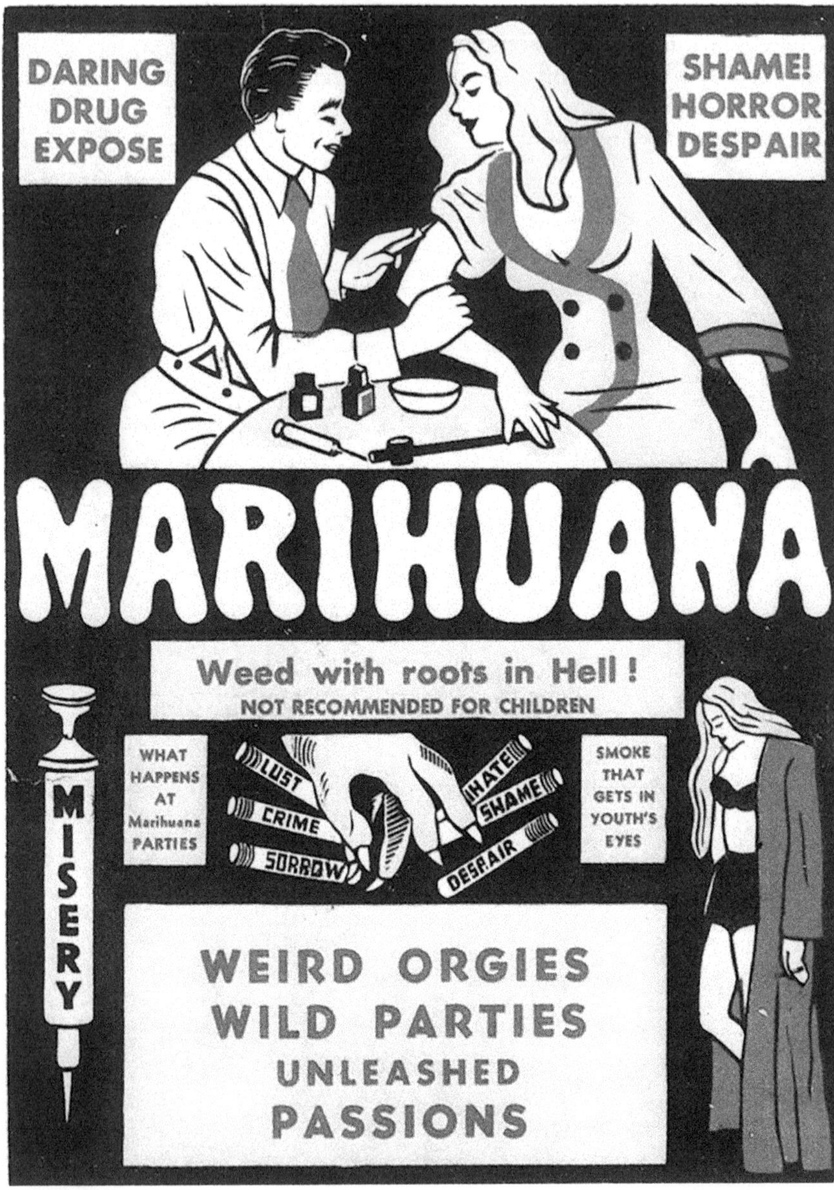
DARING
DRUG
EXPOSE
SHAME!
HORROR
DESPAIR
MARIHUANA
Weed with roots in Hell !
NOT RECOMMENDED FOR CHILDREN
WHAT
HAPPENS
AT
Marihuana
PARTIES
LUST
CRIME
SORROW
HATE
SHAME
DESPAIR
SMOKE
THAT
GETS IN
YOUTH'S
EYES
MISERY
WEIRD ORGIES
WILD PARTIES
UNLEASHED
PASSIONS

Figures 5.2a and 5.2b (Continued)

These images play ambiguously with the dual position of women, that is, as victim or enemy, in discourses on drugs. Primarily presented as a victim of drugs, seduced by men into using them (in *Marihuana* (1934) women appear as being injected by men or having their reefer lit by them projecting an

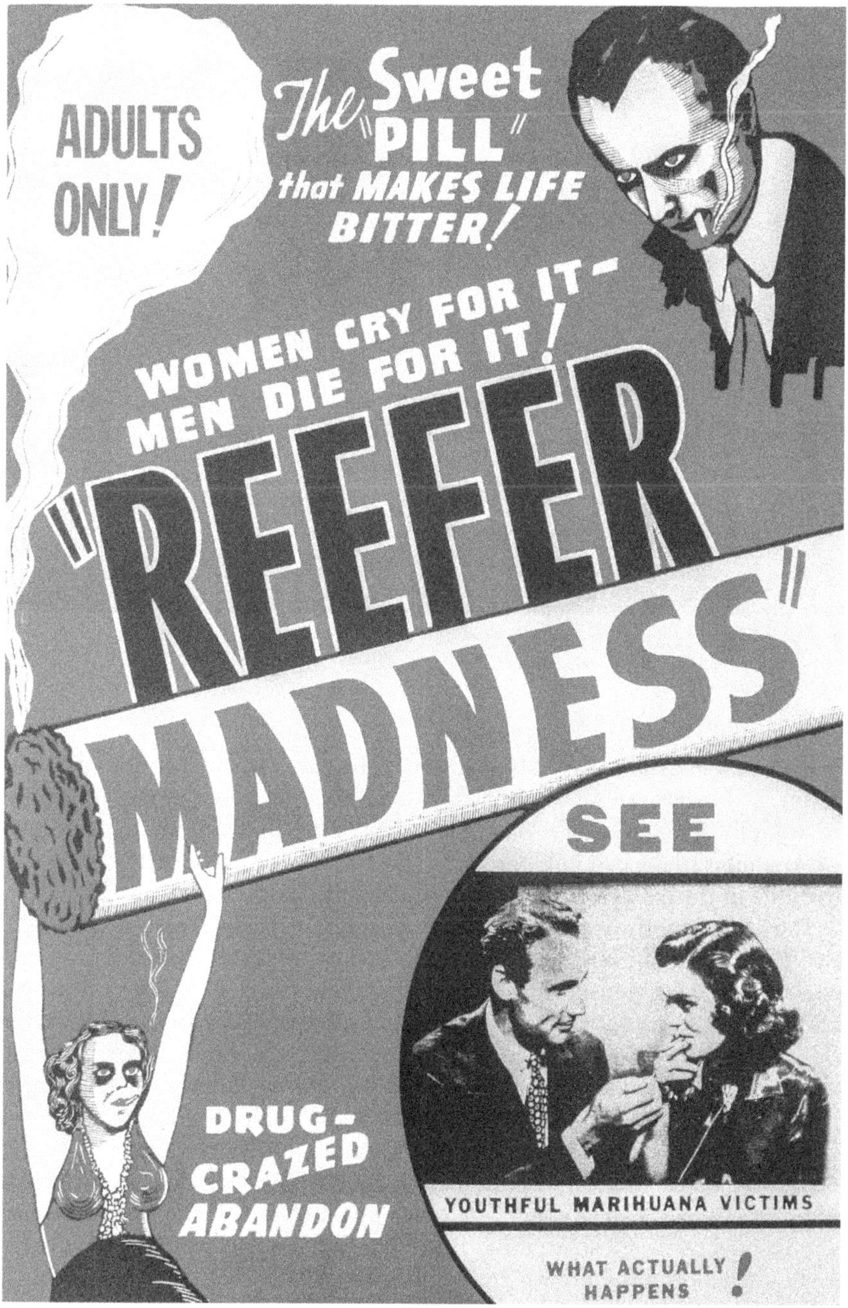
ADULTS ONLY!
The Sweet "PILL" that MAKES LIFE BITTER!
WOMEN CRY FOR IT –
MEN DIE FOR IT!
"REEFER MADNESS"
SEE
DRUG-CRAZED ABANDON
YOUTHFUL MARIHUANA VICTIMS
WHAT ACTUALLY HAPPENS!

Figures 5.3a and 5.3b *Reefer Madness* (1938)

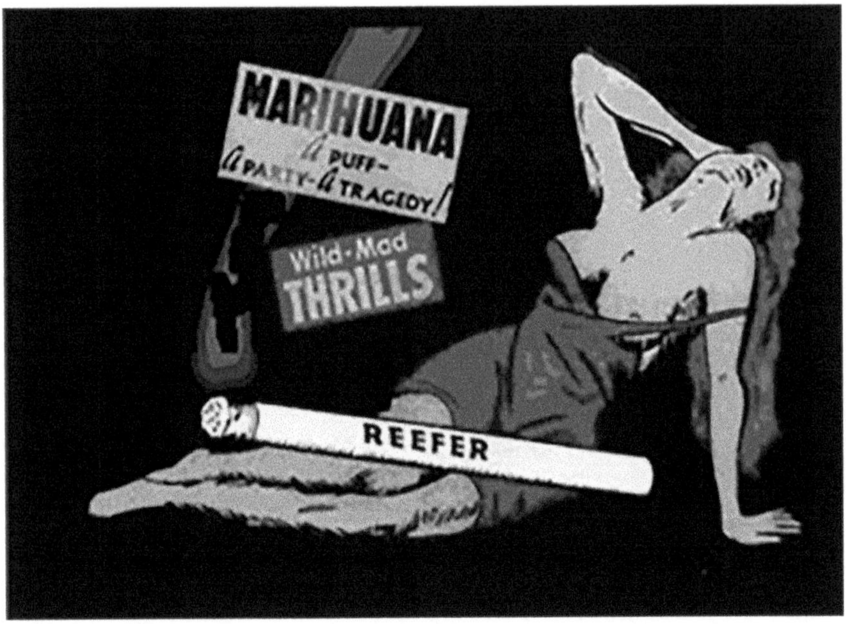

Figures 5.3a and 5.3b (Continued)

image of them as infantile, also supported by the text "youthful marihuana victim"), they are presented as a threat, seen as the fallen woman. Further, the vampire style of *Reefer Madness* produces a dehumanised image of drug users, similar to the evil in Figure 5.1. This could be thought of as a racialised overtone in the discursive context of women as victims of drugs.

The depiction of woman as a 'threat' is often made employing a sexualised gaze and portraying them as 'prostitutes' or as 'sexually available'. A moralistic overtone is present in the message of these movies, in *Reefer Madness* (1938): 'the sweet pill that makes life bitter' (first seduced then caught up in a circle of vice), 'drug crazed abandon', 'Marihuana – a puff, a party, a tragedy', 'wild-mad thrills'. In *Marihuana* (1934): 'Devil's Harvest' – 'The Smoke of Hell', 'weird orgies, wild parties, unleashed passion' accompanied by the words 'misery', 'shame, horror, despair', 'weed with roots in hell'. In Brazil, the movie *Maconha Erva Maldita* (1949) by Raul Roulien depicts, alongside other stereotypes (black people, migrants, upper class), a naïve young woman who is seduced by a lesbian drug dealer. Marihuana was seen as a trigger for crime, addiction, prostitution and homosexuality (Zanatto, 2016).

It is interesting to note how the anti-drug message of these exploitation movies seems to operate in a rather ambiguous way. While they depict women as the main victim of drugs based on the idea of moral degradation, 'a good girl until she lights a reefer', these images are used to attract audience, presenting a seductive and fetishised image of women and (of) drugs.

Discourses of women and drugs

These images still reinforce discourses surrounding women in the field of drugs, often related to traditional female social roles mainly concerning reproduction and caring for children, husband and family. These are reflected in two antagonistic images, those of the 'mother' and the 'prostitute'. The discursive dynamics of women's drug taking explicitly or implicitly circulate around sexual concerns, wherein the (culturally masculine) gaze in relation to women is (hetero) sexually oriented. It is relevant to look at how these images operate in specific contexts and the common discursive framework related to drugs in Western countries. In this sub-section, we will be focusing on the interviews conducted in Brazil.

Foucault's (1991) notion of the normative gaze refers to a surveillance that qualifies, classifies and punishes. Such practices establish over individuals a 'visibility through which one differentiates them and judges them' (p. 184). Feminist studies argue that the social and moral boundaries are more defined for women than for men, making women more visible when they transgress them. The interplay between gender, sexuality, race, age and class is understood within the dynamics of (in)visibility in public space.

The invisible domestic use of drugs, for example the use of alcohol or tranquilisers, has specific effects, particularly for women. Discourses on the invisible woman (e.g. on tranquilisers) are often of dependent, passive, victims of drugs, contrasting with the hiper-visibility of women who take drugs in public, traditionally seen as 'polluted' who have rejected their femininity (Ettorre, 1989), evoking the sexualised discourse of 'prostitution', 'sexual availability' or 'lesbianism' (aggressiveness).

This sexualised gaze could frequently be observed in the extracts from the interviews from my PhD thesis. In the following extract, S.[4] shows a discursive shift from deviant behaviour to sexual deviance:

> S. I think that there is a bit of what has in the man, in a level, but there is a whole macho (*machista*) side in relation to women, that she is a slut (*piranha*), that is willing (*que é dada*), anyway, not trustworthy, who wants to go out (*namorar*) with a woman who takes drugs? She could get mad (*pode pirar*), she could do anything, have sex with other people (*sair dando para outro*), I think that there a lot of this. . . . two people: a junkie man (*drogado*), a junkie woman, I won't make today any distinction between them, I am saying how people see it, for me both have the same disease and both have to be treated, but I think that society sees it in this way, . . ., I think that people will see the woman in a worse light (*vão ver mais mal*) more stoned (destroyed) (*detonada*) than the man, he won't be as discriminated against as she will.

In this account, the stigmatisation of women and drugs, as well as the sexual connotations stand out, as 'getting mad/high' is equated with having sex: 'she is a slut'.

Sexual deviance and madness

The way social expectations of women overlap with a sexualised position is relevant here, as female deviance is typically seen as deviating from sexual norms. In this way, it is interesting to note the sexualised connotation in gender performance in relation to drugs. Jacobson (1981) observes that for boys, cigarette smoking is also part of the expected image for them. 'It is an image that says: "I'm cool and daring; I've had sexual experience"' (p. 41), in contrast to women, who are expected to be 'quiet, demure and cooperative' (p. 41). These aspects were also emphasised by the interviewees. There W.[5] stressed the idea of women drug users as having 'mental issues', making a claim regarding the recognition of women's pleasure:

> W. You know how it is (*é daquele jeito assim*), if the guy wants to hook up with many girls (*se o cara quer catar varias minas*) he's hot (*o gostoso*), he's the big shot (*bam bam bam*), . . ., if a girls dates (*fica*) many (*vários*) guys, she's a slut (*galinha*). If the girl uses cocaine, she is because there's something wrong with her, if the guy does it he's cool (*malandro*), you get it? The guy can snort, the girl can't, if the girl snorts it is because there is something wrong with her, and it is not always like that, the girl snorts because she likes it, it isn't because she was depressive, she needed something to forget something (*do barato*), and so she went and got addicted to cocaine (*viciou*), that isn't it, she tried it (*conheceu*), liked it and got addicted (*viciou*). We don't know many things, didn't we learn to drive, to ride motorbike? . . . . Then mano,[6] I got to know (*conheci*) cocaine, I liked it, got addicted (viciei). . . . So you know (*é daquele jeito né mano*), if the guy uses it, it's because he's edgy (*ele é malandro né pá*), if the girl uses it, no, it's because she's unhinged (*doidona*), crazy (*doida*), you got it (*entendeu*)?

The association between drug taking and madness, or psychological problems for women, is evident here, as well as the analogy cited by W. comparing sexual experience and drug taking, in which for men sexual experience and drug taking are regarded as positive qualities ('smart'), while women are seen as sexually available ('slut'), or 'there is something wrong with her' ('mad'). These extracts illustrate the paradoxical ways discourses of 'madness' and 'badness' work in relation to gender. In this interview, W. points out differences in discourse about men and women drug users and defies this discursive positioning.

The way that social expectations of women interplay with a sexualised position is relevant here, as female deviance is typically seen as deviance from sexual roles. In this way, it is interesting to note the sexualised connotation in gender performances in relation to drugs. Jacobson (1981) points out that for boys cigarette smoking is also part of the image expected from them. 'It is an image that says: "I'm cool and daring; I've had sexual experience"' (p. 41), in opposition to women, who are expected to be 'quiet, demure and cooperative' (p. 41). These aspects were also emphasised by the interviewees, as seen in the interview with W., opposing to the discourse of women drug users as having 'mental issues', W. makes a claim on the recognition of women's pleasure.

The association between drug taking and madness, or psychological problems for women, was pointed out, as well as the analogy cited by W. comparing sexual experiences and drug taking, in which for men sexual experience and drug taking are regarded as good qualities ('smart), while women are seen as sexually available ('bitch), or 'there is something wrong with her' ('mad'). These extracts illustrate the paradoxical ways discourses of 'madness' and 'badness' work in relation to gender. In this interview, W. points out differences in discourse about men and women drug users and defies this discursive positioning.

Women's empowerment and tobacco industries

Within this space of moral symbolisation, it is expected for women to be in control, such that pleasure is understood as a transgressive category for women. Drug taking, in this sense, can constitute a double transgression, that is, self-indulgence and the added immorality related to drug use. Moreover, it is relevant to highlight that, due to this limited space for pleasure, the image of women and specific drugs was also explored as an empowering position. For example, in Britain during the 1920s, important changes were taking place in society, with women beginning to appear in public without the company of men and starting to smoke in public. Smoking here could be regarded as challenging the public image of women, in which 'a "public woman" was a prostitute' (Kohn, 1992, p. 52).

Hence, it is relevant to note how the image of emancipated women (who take drugs) overlaps ambivalently with sexuality. This can be seen in the next extract of J.:[7]

> J. I think that the possible difference here is the effect of the moralistic imaginary, that expects that a woman should act like this or like that and if she doesn't, she will fall into this or that social stereotype, of the slut, or of the modern woman, of the irresponsible.

It is within this moral space that notably, current cigarette ads draw on, depicting women as modern, free, daring and with power to choose and challenge traditional social stereotypes. Tobacco companies used advertisements based on themes such as power, freedom and choice, where smoking functions as a rejection of stereotypical images of women, such that 'they can be as rebellious, daring and anti-establishment as boys' (Jacobson, 1981, p. 41).

I analysed images from cigarette ad campaigns (1990s) in previous work (Mountian, 2005, 2013a), where ads targeting women frequently made use of themes of power and transgression. However, while power was observed operating in several ways, women were still portrayed through a sexualised (male) gaze. Here, I outline some of the issues arising from this analysis. Firstly, it is important to consider the advertisement's setting (both that of the image and the country of the campaign). Although I cannot further discuss the context of the ads here, it was observed that traditional 'masculine' spaces were often depicted, such as snooker halls and male locker rooms, which could be acting as an entry into a masculine world. Winston cigarette (South Africa), for example, portrayed a woman taking a shower in a male locker room with the phrase 'Do I look shy?'.

Second, messages on defying shyness, daring, emancipation, choice and freedom were emphasised. For example in the Virginia Slims '*Busca tua Verdade*' ad campaign (United States, Latina magazine), the following phrases could be found: 'I am able to decide on everything *without saying a word*'.[8] Virginia Slims: 'search for your truth'. The power obtained by smoking was portrayed as a sort of liberation, in which the woman gains the ability to decide on everything, although (still) not saying a word.

Third, ads targeted a number of racial groups in diverse contexts (e.g. Camel – 'Pleasure to Burn' campaign; Virginia Slims – 'Find your Voice' campaign in the US). In some cases, they could be seen as embodying an idea of Western models of freedom and modernity, without losing their traditions and while still remaining feminine.

Fourth, it is worthwhile analysing the way gender and sexuality are portrayed, such as in the 'I choose' Lucky Strike campaign (Spain). There, the idea of power is characterised in terms of the individual as active agent (despite the discursive tension between the idea of a lucky strike and choice). Here power to choose appears in two ways: first, the choice to smoke cigarettes (a notion that is usually under dispute in anti-tobacco campaigns that argue that smokers are addicted, and therefore, not free); and second, the active role of choosing in other daily life contexts, such as sexual partners, with both heterosexual and homosexual partners being depicted in this campaign. When analysing these images, it was also possible to see antagonistic conceptions of women and cigarettes (drugs), although smoking is portrayed as liberating and as challenging stereotypical female roles, the images were produced from a specific perspective, positioning and depicting women via a sexualised gaze.

5.3 Drug policy, gender, sexuality and race

These stereotypical images on the intersections between gender, sexuality, race, class, age and disability, can frequently be found operating in the context of drug policies, often. The analysis of the dynamics of the normative gaze and the discursive position of the 'other' in relation to women and drugs can provide relevant insights for intervention and research settings.

> Medical and psychological literature presented a picture of drug use in which drug users just happened to be male and women hardly figured. When they did, they appeared as sicker, more deviant, more psychologically disturbed than their male peers: as weak and pathetic creatures. Women's drug use figured as a 'deviation' from 'normal' femininity due to mental or physical deficiencies, or disease.
>
> (Henderson, 1999, p. 37)

Regarding the particular discursive position of women, it is notable how drug treatment for women is frequently tackled in light of how their drug use affected others, that is childbirth, child rearing and sexual activities. In this manner, the HIV epidemic has had a significant impact on services for women drug users, leading to a growth in policy-led research. As Campbell (2000, p. 25) argues, drug use is understood as a 'form of violence that women commit against themselves and those closest to them'. Women's health or illness is often connected to the idea of harming others, where prostitution, pregnancy and childcare become crucial dimensions. The focus on the transmission of disease to others can also be seen in policies for *travestis* and transwomen and male prostitution.

During the 90's, stereotypical images of women drug users could be seen once again circulating in the media (for example crack-mothers). Campbell analysed the effects of these images in public policies (such as punitive actions):

> While in the past women addicts who were pregnant or mothering were constructed as poor mothers who violated feminine norms by dominating their households, in the latter decades of the century women who biologically 'reproduced' addiction played stunningly demonised roles.
>
> (Campbell, 2000, p. 139)

These discourses are based on the idea that women drug users cannot control themselves and, therefore, cannot educate their children, and thus will – given women's roles in relation to nation – contribute to (re)producing an unruly society.

During the 1980s and 90s, policy makers drew on the idea of the 'vulnerable child' or the 'foetus' positioning women either as victims or 'victimisers', and thereby deciding on either a punitive or therapeutic approach for drug policy. This created two possible policy options: either the expansion of the health and social apparatus or a punitive legal approach. A key discourse identified in this context was the 'decline of the maternal instinct' as the source of the problem (Campbell, 2000), and as such, there was a call for public surveillance, in which each citizen acquires the moral obligation to prevent mothers or future mothers from taking drugs, which can also put women's autonomy over their bodies and lives in jeopardy.

Here, an individualistic approach is adopted, wherein society, including the father, is exempted from any responsibility. Indeed, the social isolation of women drug users increases during pregnancy, creating a different set of problems (Klee et al., 2002). The social stigma and the possibility of having their children taken away by government authorities can operate as an obstacle for women to seek help when necessary, increasing *invisibility* and social isolation.

Another key issue in the field of gender and drugs regards domestic violence against women and drug use (e.g. alcohol) by men. This calls for an analysis that considers how violence against women operates in society. McDonald (1994) highlights how behaviour is learnt, and as such drunken behaviour is also learnt. In this sense, physical abuse due to alcohol consumption is socially and culturally located. It is important to note that drug policy is driven by a 'law and order' agenda, which also appears to have a public/private split in that drug policies are chiefly concerned with criminality and violence on the streets rather than in the domestic sphere. Therefore, violence against women in the home when it is linked to substance abuse is frequently overlooked. In this way the development of services and treatments that consider the specificities of women and LGBTQI+ people and the social context is vital.

Brazilian context and drug policies

In the Brazilian context,[9] in terms of social and political dimensions, it is important to emphasise that despite being one of the largest global economies, Brazil ranks 12th in social inequality (Soares, 2013). The rates of violence and homicide are extremely high, particularly in relation to the black population (IPEA, 2021), and black adolescents (Cerqueira & Coelho IPEA, 2017). It is the 5th most violent country for women, particularly black women, out of 83 countries (Waiselfisz, 2015), and with high rates of sexual violence against women (Maito et al., 2021), in addition to high rates of violence against the lesbian, gay, bisexual, *travesti* and transsexual (LGBTTQIA+) populations (TGEU, 2016; Benevides & Nogueira, 2021).

Brazil has a large incarcerated population (in absolute numbers, it has the third-largest incarcerated population globally), showing a 74% increase during the period from 2005 to 2012, jumping from 296,919 to 514,482 detainees, with 60.8% being black and 25.3% (in 2012) imprisoned for drug-related issues (Brazil, 2015). In 2019, there were more than 750,000 detainees (INFOPEN, 2019). There was an increase in the number of adolescents serving custodial sentences, from 19,595 in 2011 to 20,532 in 2012, with 27% being for drug-related crimes (Waiselfisz, 2015).

The female prison population also grew, being the fifth largest in the world (absolute numbers). Between 2000 and 2014, it grew 567%, surpassing the increase in male incarceration (119%), totalling 37,380 women in prison, with 68% being for drug-related crimes. The majority of the female prison population is composed of black women (68%), about half are between 18 and 29 years old, half never completed elementary education (INFOPEN, 2016; Ormeño, 2012), 81% have children and are the main or sole providers for their families, usually without having previous criminal records (ITTC, 2015). However, prison infrastructure was not planned for women nor for LGBTQI+people, and issues associated with maternity among others stand out. The stigma of imprisoned women is significant, noticeable in the small number of women who receive prison visits in comparison to male prisons. It is crucial to consider the way that gender, race and class intersect in drug policies in Brazil, as well as how the black population is affected, regarding homicide, imprisonment and drug-related sentences.[10]

Analysing drug policies in Brazil – which in practice are primarily based on absenteeism and punitivist conceptions – we can highlight that, as an effect, there is a lack of information about drugs, putting at risk the health of people who use them, a lack of research and data, an increase in incarceration (Karam, 2007; Lemgruber et al., 2021) and in violence and homicide, and an increase in stigma and discrimination related to drug users. This can be seen for example in the way that crack users are commonly referred to as 'zombies', or '*noias*'.[11] Further, it is essential to consider the removal of children from women drug users without proper evaluation or social support, which occurs particularly among poor, black women (Malheiro, 2020), as well as public policies for pregnant women (Macedo et al., 2021).

Moreover, the dynamics of invisibility of drug use by women in isolation and greater ostracism is important to be accounted for in health policy, as having specific effects and pointing to obstacles for women to seek assistance when needed. Research, public programs and most drug-related public policy, including the legal institution, were traditionally based on male, heterosexual experience (as seen elsewhere Margo, 2016); therefore, awareness of gender, sexuality, race, class, age and disability becomes crucial.

Another key aspect is how sexuality is considered in the field of drugs. Firstly, it is important to consider the effects of LGBTphobia on individuals, as well as the structural reproduction of this violence in institutions and public policy. Drug-related public policy frequently overlooks issues surrounding sexuality, creating the risk of silencing and marginalising these populations. Therefore, beyond the relative lack of initiatives that consider the specificities of these groups (Ettorre, 2005), several reports found that institutions, including health institutions, stigmatise LGBTQI+ people, who suffer, in addition to insults and inadequate service, disrespect to their adopted name (nome social),[12] which represents an obstacle for this population to access health services. Furthermore, additional research is needed regarding the well-being of LGBTQI+ people placed in religious-based drug treatment centres, called 'therapeutic communities' in Brazil (Santos, 2018).

Other important points for our consideration include analysing the hypersexualisation and social devaluation of LGBTTQI+ people, wherein, similarly to discourses on drug users, they have traditionally been seen as deviant, sinful and/or mentally ill. These discourses have an effect on public policy, particularly when there is a stigmatising discursive association between this group and drug abuse, tapping into historical discourses (Masur & Carlini, 1994), as seen in Chapter 2.

Regarding the specificities of these groups, it is essential to recognise the effects of LGBTphobia considering the intersectional relations present in this context, such as obstacles when accessing health services, the lack of research on the specificities of drug use by LGBTTQI+ people and the lack of public policy that considers the specificities of this population, particularly for trans people, *travestis*, transgender and transexual people. All these considerations should be re-calibrated to think about harm reduction strategies, considering that, in many cases, there is also the use of other substances such as hormones, etc. (Mountian, 2015a).

It is also important to critically analyse the drug use of cisgender women and LGBTQI+ people and the cases of violence against them. It is fundamental to socially and culturally locate the violence, that is, the structural context that allows it to occur. As we have seen, rates of violence against women and LGBTQI+ people in Brazil are extremely high, both in cases of sexual violence and homicide (TGEU, 2016). Additionally, the high suicide rate among the LGBTQI+ population (seen in research as a response to the prejudice they suffer (Tosh, 2016)) also needs to be considered. Given the social context, taking into account the social dimensions of race, class and age, harm reduction policies are crucial to assess the risks that cisgender women are exposed to in sexist environments, as well as the risks that LGBTQI+ people suffer in homophobic, transphobic and LGBTQphobic settings.

Final considerations

In this chapter, we sought to analyse the social imaginary surrounding women and drugs, looking at key discourses on drug use and how these operate in relation to gender. This is particularly relevant to understand how these discourses mobilise tropes of 'dependency', 'weakness', 'uncontrollability' and 'madness', characteristics commonly associated with drug use and drug users that are also seen as feminine characteristics, and that serve to locate the position of the Other. From this, we saw how the sexualised gaze operates in relation to women, where specific binary discourses such as the 'bad mother', the 'prostitute' or the rejection of femininity (pejoratively referred to 'lesbians') are reproduced.

The limiting scope of these discourses is also connected to the position of women in terms of the nation. Understood as the guardians of society's morality, drug use is seen as a special threat for women, their children and the nation at large. Thus, within the binary logic that maps out the coordinates of this moral framework, women are portrayed as either the primary victims or perpetrators of drug use.

This imaginary position is further clarified by the notion of the gaze, given that the dynamics of visibility and invisibility of women and drugs are driven by a (sexualised) gaze, either through the invisible use of drugs at home; or the hyper visibility of drug taking (including alcohol) in public. Furthermore, due to this limited discursive space available for indulgence, drug taking was also viewed as a challenge to social norms (public woman x woman in public). However, in our analysis of cigarette campaigns, we also saw how this possible space of empowerment was exploited by the tobacco industry, as well as mobilising contradictory and antagonistic discourses that establish stereotypical social roles.

When drafting drug public policy, it is vital that we consider these analyses of the social imaginary surrounding women, in addition to the intersectional social categories of race, sexuality, age and class. In these examples, we can see how drug policies are often informed by an implicit moral foundation and are intrinsically related to how minoritised groups are socially viewed. It is important to emphasise that the effects of these policies operate differently depending on the context, generating different outcomes in producer and consumer countries (Souza, 2015; Mountian, 2017c).

It is fundamental for drug policies to become sensitive to LGBTQI+ and women-oriented issues (Ettorre, 1989; Raine, 2001), reflecting an awareness of the relations between gender, sexuality, race, age, disability and class, within a framework that includes women and LGBTQI+ people as social actors. This intersectional character (related to gender, sexuality, race, age, disability and class) should also be further expanded to encompass current gaps in policy and provision.

Notes

1 K. female, white, 48 years old, mother of 3 children, in Public Hospital for treatment for alcohol, unemployed
2 Idiomatic expression
3 Exploitation movies focused on sensational themes, such as drug abuse, prostitution and venereal disease, among others. These movies are regarded as responsible for the survival of independent movie theatres across U.S. (Feaster & Wood, interviewed by Johnson, 2004).
4 Male, White, 28 years old, in treatment for drug use
5 Female, Black, 25 years old, student, in treatment for drug use
6 Idiomatic expression
7 Male, White, 28 years old, businessman
8 Translated by the author
9 Based on the book chapter (Mountian, 2017c)
10 http://ibccrim.jusbrasil.com.br/noticias/2569562/trafico-de-drogas
11 Pejorative term, deriving from paranoia
12 Name chosen by the individual

Conclusion

Decolonising mental health

This book explores the diverse social power dynamics active in the inclusion/exclusion of minoritised groups in mental health theory and practice, and their role in the production of subjectivity, subject positions, identity and desire. While I provide some resources for health and mental health service providers, the main objective was to analyse the production and maintenance of the position of the Other in the area of mental health. By deconstructing the position of the Other, I highlighted the production of a therapeutic culture, aiming to outline other possibilities for mental health frameworks and, crucially, to challenge the Us-Other divide, thereby opening up discursive spaces for the emergence of alternative subject positions, that is, beyond simply the position of the Other.

The debates considered here highlight current and historical understandings of mental health research and practice, particularly focusing on the importance of understanding social context and the intersections between gender, sexuality, race, class, age and disability, for a critical analysis of the production of psy-theory and practice. These issues become evident in the interaction between health practitioners and service users, affecting both treatment and research.

There are a number of important aspects involving the relationship between otherness and mental health highlighted in the research conducted that are worth us considering. These include the clear need observed in studies on immigrants and mental health, for an ongoing *reflexivity* on the part of the practitioner and researcher regarding the relational/transferential position of the professional, rethinking pre-conceived ideas on immigrants and about how discourses on culture, race and gender operate. Given the importance of avoiding an over hasty pathologisation of subjects and a mental health framework based on the idea of isolated individuals divested of a broader social context, it is essential to consider immigration and settlement processes, as well as the diverse perspectives and knowledge on mental health of immigrants.

From the studies into drug addiction and women, two main aspects were emphasised: firstly, the moral issues involved in the production of the notion of drug addiction, which produces a particular discursive space surrounding processes of othering, and, within this, secondly, the role of gender, sexuality, race and age in research and treatment, that is, how specific groups are affected by stigmatising and criminalising perspectives surrounding drugs, such as the effects of stigmatisation on women and LGBTQI+ people, and the criminalisation of young black men and women (in Brazil), and other minoritised groups. Women and LGBTQI+ people are still marginalised in research, as drug treatment and research were traditionally designed for men, which can also operate as an obstacle for seeking help when needed, particularly when there is a lack of adequate environment in services for LGBTQI+ people and women, and a risk of losing the guardianship of children.

Finally, in the analysis of othering processes, the effects of mental health categories related to sexuality must be clearly apprehended, as homosexuality and transsexuality were seen as mental health disorders *per se*. From the research conducted with older *travestis* and transgender women in Brazil, the lack of awareness of the specificities of these populations on the part of health services, such as the effects of transphobic experiences, body changes and ageing, became clear. At the same time, transphobic practices in health services themselves reported by the participants were experienced as a further barrier to treatment. These aspects hinder the access of trans people to health and mental health care services. Therefore, it is crucial to consider the specificities of trans people, and the effects of transphobia and homophobia on the subject for mental health research and care, given the impact of violence on mental health. We must also critically analyse the reproductions of othering processes seen in the analysis of social-historical pathologising views of transsexuality and homosexuality.

The issues raised in this book seek to inform the debate around a growing awareness of processes of othering, emphasising the importance of considering the subject's social context and the intersections between gender, race, class, age, disability and sexuality. That is, how primitivising (working class), orientalising (immigrant) and sexualising (gender and sexuality) discursive strands operate in relation to subjectivity and mental health perspectives. Given this, we defended the need for an ongoing critical *reflexivity* on the part of the researcher and the practitioner in relation to any pre-conceived notions regarding the Other. This requires a continuing awareness of the researcher's position in listening to the subject. From this, key insights concerning the encounter between the subject and mental health provider were gleaned, firstly, regarding the position of the Other (re)produced within these encounters, and secondly, in terms of how to provide alternative discursive spaces to be able to listen to the Other, more specifically, for the emergence of the subject.

The reflexivity of the researcher is crucial when developing research. Although we cannot go into this further in this manuscript, in all research we undertook different challenges and outcomes presented themselves from the researcher/subject encounter, which necessitated the adoption of diverse strategies. I will present further details in the next section and in appendix 1.

In the first part of the book, I explored the key theoretical perspectives utilised. In Chapter 1, the epistemological framework adopted throughout the manuscript and for our research was outlined, highlighting the key conceptualisations on the intersectionality of race, gender, class, age and disability. Consideration of these categories was seen as fundamental for both research and practice, while also seeking to avoid essentialising the subject into them. We also argued for the importance of accounting for the social context for an effective critical analysis of mental health theory and praxis.

Chapter 2 provided a historical perspective on psychiatric diagnosis and how it affects specific minoritised groups, focusing on women and the association with hysteria and depression; immigration and the effects on mental health; on the diagnosis of homosexuality and transsexuality; and on the history of addiction and intersections with gender, race and class. There are intertwined relations between diagnostics and othering processes, which, on one hand, can emphasise the constraints that minoritised group experience, while, on the other hand, highlights how Othered groups can be discursively positioned as pathological, as seen in the case of LGBTQI+ people, women, immigrants and ethnic minoritised communities.

The second part of the book presented the results of our research. In Chapter 3, a number of issues surrounding mental health and immigration were explored, including the importance of a culturally sensitive approach, translation services, being aware of the hardships of migratory processes (war, uncertainty, effects of sexism, xenophobia and racism, adaptation, bureaucratic difficulties, social isolation) and access to health services (information on how to access health services, and material on prevention in different languages, including drug use). Pre-conceived notions of immigrants, refugees and asylum seekers can affect both the theory and practice of mental health and health care, such as in ideas of immigrants bringing disease to the country, idealised images of motherhood which do not necessarily correspond to immigrant experience, and the culturally diverse understandings of health and mental health.

It is also essential that we consider the diversity of understandings of mental health, as immigrants can be the object of overly hasty diagnoses. Concomitantly, the situatedness of psy-knowledge also needs to be called into question, that is, the acknowledgement of the social and historical context of the production of knowledge and practice. In the research conducted, while these aspects were highlighted as obstacles for accessing health services, in some contexts, health service providers showed knowledge and engagement with immigrants, such that a dialogue between the service user and provider resulted in a sense of the health centre as a safe space for the immigrant. Moreover, there are differences both between types of service, and between services in the UK and in Brazil, mostly related to resource shortfalls. In this case, it is worthwhile noting the effort of some service providers to overcome such issues.

The results of the various studies on immigration cited here were based on a range of research collaborations and data collection strategies. For example, in the research on drug use and young asylum seekers in the UK, it was a service provider who interviewed the other service providers. In the research on access to health services in Manchester, the fieldwork consisted of individual interviews and focus groups organised by a group of stakeholders from immigrant community organisations. The fieldwork was carried out by a male native researcher and by a female researcher who was an immigrant in the context. In the research conducted in Brazil, part of the fieldwork was based on workshops for health service providers run by the immigrants themselves.

Chapter 4 emphasised the effects of structural transphobia on access to basic rights and its effects on health and mental health theory and treatment. This is based on interviews with older *travestis* in Brazil and on research on trans people's access to education. The fieldwork for this study was carried out by a transwoman and cisgender people who work in the educational field and policy makers.

Anyky Lima (2012) pointed out that 'most *travestis* are marginal all their lives and when they get old, they become old marginals (*marginais*)'. This is the starting point for our research, that is, the marginalisation of *travestis* in Brazil. Transphobia was observed from childhood, being expelled from schools, family and communities, with many *travestis* experiencing exclusion and institutional vulnerability. Campaigns against homophobia and transphobia were implemented although face resistance from traditional religious groups and government sectors (Correa et al., 2021). The interviews with older *travestis* uncovered stories stretching from the era of the military dictatorship to the period of democratisation. During the military dictatorship, violence from the police and the army was common, together with street violence, which continues up to the present, as rates of assault and homicide against *travestis* and trans people in Brazil remain high. Immigration to safer environments was seen as a possibility for security and social mobility. Old age for this population, which probably is younger than that for the rest the Brazilian population, shows the non-inclusion of trans people in health services, which often overlooked bodily changes in this demographic. Older age also reduced the already limited employment possibilities, such that some *travestis* masculinise in order to find work. The stories of *travestis* and trans people in Brazil show the effects of transphobic contexts and the need for awareness of the intersectional categories of gender, race, class, age and disability in health services and public policy.

Chapter 5 based on my doctoral research on gender and drug use highlighted how the intersections between gender, race, class and age operate within conceptions of drug use, drug addiction and drug policy. The interviews were conducted by the researcher in in-treatment locations as well as informal settings. The position of the researcher, who is also a psychologist, might have triggered specific answers from the participants who were in-patients. This was analysed in terms of the medical discourses in which drug use is embedded. The discursive position of women in discourses surrounding drug use was twofold. On one hand, it drew on a stereotyped image of women as infantile, vulnerable and dependent, while, on the other, it projected a hypersexualised gaze towards women, reifying the moralising figure of the fallen woman. At the same time, treatment and research also failed to account for LGBTQI+ people, thereby showing an insensitivity towards the needs of diverse minority communities. These images frequently present in research and treatment contexts can have a significant impact, showing the importance of considering gender, sexuality and the intersections with race, age, class and disability for health services.

From these studies, we can observe the way that Othering processes permeate health practices. The close relationship between minoritised groups and diagnostics and the need to consider the social context and structural discourses on intersectional categories for analysis become evident. Given this, we can, on one hand, interrogate how psy-disciplines can reproduce these specific discourses and, on the other hand, examine how we can listen to the Other, which I will further elaborate here, focusing on the effects of medical diagnoses. The way that specific ideas operate within medical and psychological practice and the (re)production of these discourses in diagnostics must be critically interrogated. Indeed, as Fernando (2012) argues, diagnosis becomes part of the problem in relation to 'ethnic' issues, with a critical approach to the model of mental illness being crucial, particularly regarding our understanding of 'illness'.

It is necessary that we highlight some issues for critical analysis, firstly the recognition of the intersectional dynamics of the social categories and how they interpellate the subject, without essentialising or reifying the subject. Second, the importance of assessing how these social categories operate in health and mental health discourses and institutions, and thirdly, the analysis of the encounters between the subject and psy-professionals, situating psy-disciplines and deconstructing preconceived notions of the Other.

The importance of considering how the key social categories operate in health and mental health services has been highlighted throughout this manuscript, as well as possibilities of resisting and enlarging the supposedly static positions given to these social groups, which is an ongoing challenge for both practical and theoretical contexts. As previously noted, numerous authors, including Gonzalez (2020), Fanon (1986), Said (1978), Kilomba (2019), Bhabha (1994), Lorde (1984), Hooks (1984), Ahmed (2012), McClintock (1995), Gilroy (2000), Hall (2008), Sedgwick (1991), among many others, have debated the effects of the homogenised views on minoritised groups. The way that intersectional categories of race, gender, sexuality, class, age, and disability operate within society and in health and mental health areas has also been critically analysed (Burman & Chantler, 2003; Fernando, 2012; Littlewood & Lipsedge, 1989; Mills, 2014), and a number of strategies have been developed, such as the use of monitoring systems for social categories. Fernando (2012) highlights the use of monitoring for ethnicity, culture and race for service planning in order to identify discrimination and overcome social injustice; however, without fixing this identification to the subject, 'ethnic identity should not be made into an over-arching part of how we see ourselves as individuals, it is not DNA. It is just one of the many diverse aspects of the "self"' (Fernando, 2012, pp. 119–120).

It is crucial, therefore, not to reduce the subject to a category, but rather to consider the structures that produce these categories and how they interpellate the subjects. It is within constitutive encounters that the position of the Other is produced, and in this sense, I have investigated the possibilities for discursive renewal available within such encounters. As with conceptions about race, gender and sexuality, culture is a fluid category, and as such, it is through the deconstruction of the historical fixity of specific repeating signifiers that possibilities for opening alternative positions for the Other can be envisaged.

Regarding alternative discursive spaces, it is relevant to note the debates surrounding hybridity and in-betweenness, such as Anzaldúa's (1987) reflections on the *mestiza*. In this sense, it is questioned how ambivalence and hybridity can offer alternative discursive frameworks for subjects and diverse social dynamics. As Mills (2014) points out:

> In Bhabha's ambivalence and hybridity, a different space is opened, a space where differences between cultures are not accommodated – a 'third space' (Rutherford, 1990) . . . . This hints at other ways of conceptualizing difference within GMH [Global Mental Health]– for example, in encountering the 'treatment gap' not as a space to be closed through applying universal psychiatric criteria, but as a borderline, a place of hybrid understandings, that enables other ways of responding to distress to be encountered, ways that may disrupt psychiatry. This is Bhabha's (1994, p. 4) space 'in-between' that 'opens up the possibility of a cultural hybridity that entertains difference without an assumed or imposed hierarchy'. For Bhabha this is a 'third space' that sets up 'new structures of authority, new political initiatives, which are inadequately understood through received wisdom' (Rutherford, 1990, p. 211). This space to decolonize psychiatry and GMH is more than purely conceptual, for these 'new political initiatives' are already at work in a practical way in the global South.
>
> (Mills, 2014, p. 138)

Through a critical analysis of the encounter, we are able to unravel the power relations that are intrinsically part of this dynamic, opening a discursive space to challenge these fixed positions. As Ahmed highlights 'An ethics that responds to each other as if they were other in the same way is inadequate' (Ahmed, 2000, p. 16). Similarly, it is relevant to question the production of 'fixed' identities within the frame of borders. Taking up Brah's assertion (1996), the border must be contextualised:

> I have suggested before, namely that diasporic or border positionality does not *in itself* assure a vantage point of privileged insight into and understanding of relations of power, although it does create a space in which experiential mediations may intersect in ways that render such understandings more readily accessible. It is essentially a question of politics. Diasporic identities cannot be read off in a one-to-one fashion straightforwardly from a border positionality, in the same way that a feminist subject position cannot be deduced from the category 'woman'. This point deserves emphasis especially because the proliferation of discourses about 'border crossings' and 'diasporic identities' might be taken to imply a common standpoint or a universalised notion of 'border consciousness'. Rather, there are multiple semiotic spaces at diasporic borders, and the probability of certain forms of consciousness emerging are subject to the play of political power and psychic investments in the maintenance or erosion of the status quo.
>
> (Brah, 1996, p. 204)

The contextualisation of processes of Othering is fundamental for a critical rereading of the fields of health and mental health, and of how specific distinctions are produced in the encounter between services and the subject. As such, it is crucial to contextualise racialisation processes; to understand how racial/ethnic, gender and class boundaries dynamics; and to challenge practices of exclusion (Anthias & Yuval-Davis, 1996).

The analysis of the reproduction of the Other (and of boundaries) and strategies to provide space for the emergence of the subject are central aspects for decolonising practices in the fields of health and mental health. It is within this arena that the question regarding the possibilities for listening to the Other is posed.

Listening to the other: psychoanalytic contributions

> Thus, to understand a society means, first and foremost, to penetrate or reappropriate the social imaginary significations which hold this society together. Is this at all possible? We have to take into account two facts here.
>
> The first, indisputable fact is that *almost all* of the people in a given society do not and cannot understand a "foreign" society. (I am not speaking, of course, about trivial obstacles.) This points to what I have called the cognitive closure of the institution. The second (which can be and is disputed, but to which I nevertheless hold) is that under some very specific social, historical, and personal preconditions, some people can understand something about a foreign society. This points to some sort of "potential universality" in whatever is human for humans. Contrary to inherited commonplaces, the root of this universality is

> not human "rationality" (if "rationality" were at stake here, nobody would ever have had understood anything about the Hebrew God, or, for that matter, about any religion whatsoever), but creative imagination as the nuclear component of nontrivial thinking. Whatever has been imagined strongly enough to shape behavior, speech or objects can, in principle, be re-imagined (re-represented, *wiedervorgestellt*) by somebody else.
>
> (Castoriadis, 1991, p. 85)

The epistemological enclosures on listening to the Other have been debated by Spivak (1988) under the question *Can the Subaltern Speak*? From this starting point, I developed reflections around possibilities for listening. Firstly, in terms of the need for a critical reflexivity (Mountian, 2017a) in relation to the position of the researcher and practitioner. At the same time, we must seek to avoid essentialising or objectifying the Other, which can prevent the subject from speaking/being heard. Secondly, we must consider approaches that account for the Other's voice, that is, allow the subject's voice, and crucially, their desire to emerge/be heard. Questions on who can speak (Kilomba, 2019) and what are the 'things that can't be said' (Frosh, 2014) broaden the discursive spaces towards decolonial and feminist frameworks, bringing to the forefront the social context, for example in the difference between asking 'what have you done' and 'what has racism done to you' (Kilomba, 2019, p. 226). While both queries are legitimate, it is crucial that we consider how, when and for whom they are produced. The reflections proposed here focus on the possibilities for opening discursive spaces for the subject to speak, considering the subject's experience (including the effects of racism, sexism). For this, the question regarding how the Other can be heard is essential. Bhabba (1986 London, in Fanon, 1994, XXV), claiming a return to Fanon, interrogates: '[H]ow can the human world live its difference? How can a human being live Other-wise?'

These ambiguous relations are seen in various contexts and affect mental health practices with minoritised groups, as seen in the studies presented here. Here the limited discursive possibilities available to the Other are uncovered, commonly positioning them as victim or threat, and often exoticised or reified as a fetishised Other. In this sense, it was highlighted that considering relations of gender, sexuality and race is vital to our critical analysis, and a view of what the discursive possibilities available to the gendered, racialised and sexualised subject are. The discursive possibilities of the position of the Other must interrogated, for a listening that provides space for the emergence of the subject, that is, the subject of desire, able to present paradoxes and ambiguities (Badiou, 2001), and to represent themselves (Spivak, 1988).

Feminist, decolonial and anti-racist authors have reflected on the possibilities of listening to the Other, underlining the risk of reproducing fixed discursive positions for them, particularly flagging the danger of inferiorisation and pathologisation of the subject. This debate is also seen in psychoanalysis; for example, feminist psychoanalysts emphasise how sexist relations within patriarchal societies function in the construction of subjectivity, in and outside psychoanalysis (Rose, 1994; Frosh, 1995; Malone, 2006; Chodorow, 1989; Segal, 2015; Gianesi & Mountian, 2019), and post-colonial and decolonial studies point out the effects of colonial and racial relations on subjectivity (Fanon, 1986; Seshadri-Crooks, 2000; Santos, 1983). These analyses highlight the production of subjectivity, and the risks of essentialising and fetishising the subject, challenging causalistic views on the relations within theoretical perspectives. In the case of psychoanalysis, this becomes the disentangling of causal relations, for example in the relations between gender-sex-practice-desire (Butler, 1999).

Assuming these critiques, it is possible to observe certain dimensions of psychoanalytic theory that challenge these established positions and can provide an emancipatory space for subjects (see Parker, 2011). There are theoretical developments that bring insights into this field, allowing to critically revisit psychiatric diagnosis (e.g. challenging medical dominated notion of institutional trauma from a feminist standpoint (Thompson, 2021)), reviewing psychoanalytic praxis (Layton et al., 2006; Ryan, 2017) and conceptions from critical perspectives (e.g. melancholia from a Fanonian perspective (Gordon, 2007)), and the connections between psychoanalytical conceptualisations for critical analysis (social imaginary, Castoriadis, 1991). Maintaining a critical perspective on theory and therapeutic practice, we note how clinical practice, as a space for the possibility of emancipation, can provide some elements for a critical feminist and decolonial understanding of the subject, which can also expand the debate regarding the experience of the hybridity or the *mestiza* (Anzaldúa, 1987). This socially engaged perspective can be seen, for example, in the learnings from the black feminist self-care practice (based on Lorde's work (Nayak, 2020)), Fanon's clinical praxis (mental health treatment as a form of symptom, situating knowledge and practice (Gibson & Beneduce, 2019)), anti-psychiatric movements (Laing, Basaglia, Cooper, Nise da Silveira, among others) and psychoanalytic social clinics (Freud, 1918; Danto, 2019; Soreanu, 2019). Here I will focus on the debates of the psychoanalytical listening for a critical analysis.

Language is a constitutive element of subjectivity for psychoanalysis, and listening is a central issue in psychoanalytic studies and practice. From Fanon's (1986) assertion that 'to speak a language is to take on a world, a culture', it is possible to highlight the challenges posed to psychoanalysis, particularly regarding the ongoing debate about how to consider the social context and power relations when analysing the subject. This is relevant for clinical practice, as social relations and context can either be neglected or taken as a homogeneous phenomenon. Freud highlights how the social is immanent to the analysis of the subject, and Lacan further elaborates on the importance of language for the constitution of subjectivity.

> It is true that individual psychology is concerned with the individual man and explores the paths by which he seeks to find satisfaction for

> his instinctual impulses; but only rarely and under certain exceptional conditions is individual psychology in a position to disregard the relations of this individual to others. In the individual's mental life someone else is invariably involved, as a model, as an object, as a helper, as an opponent; and so from the very first individual psychology, in is extended but entirely justifiable sense of the words, is at the same time social psychology as well.
>
> (Freud, 1921, p. 2)

In further considering the dilemmas and possibilities involved in listening within a psychoanalytic framework, we find that psychoanalytic listening, sensitive to social context and the subject's desire implies an ethical perspective on the part of the psychoanalyst (or psychologist). This is manifest in an ongoing reflexivity, which also presupposes an awareness of their own position. This ethical positioning recognises the social power relations involved in the patient/therapist relationship, without assuming these as an inherent dimension of the subject, while remaining aware of the effects of social exclusion on subjectivity. This listening can allow us to set in motion connections that break up imaginary identifications while simultaneously helping us to clarify some of the subjective effects of social exclusion and power relations.

For this critical project, the consideration of the social imaginary that situates the subject is fundamental (Mountian, 2009). Rosa (1999) highlights the importance of observing the role of social imaginary in the constitution of the subject, as the discourse of the 'Other' (Lacanian Other) that is relevant to the constitution of the subject is impregnated by the imaginary production of the social group. Rosa (1998) discusses the effects of the social imaginary on homeless young people in Brazil, given that beyond poverty itself, there is a social imaginary of delinquency. As such, within the relationship between culture and subjectivity, alongside numerous other failures of protection, these young people lack a place in the social ideal, instead occupying a marginalised discursive space. The analysis includes the issue of the subject's relationship to the law, as a result of how social bonds are structured (Rosa, 1999, 2000). Therefore, it is important to investigate the fantasies expressed by social groups. Focusing on the history and place occupied by the child, it is possible to argue that these spaces produce different discourses also depending on other categories, such as gender, race and class (Burman, 2015). Addressing the importance of the imaginary, Roof (1996) underlines the difficulties involved in confronting the Law, with the distinction between its metaphorical devices and structural functions being particularly problematic, given that ideas about the Law are already imaginary, that is, are gendered and metaphorical.

Hence this framework facilitates an investigation of how social fantasies and imaginary formations inform discourses (Mountian, 2009). Work with discourse analysis can provide insights for such an approach, uncovering discursive structures and their associated effects in constituting subjectivity. Within this, a discursive analytic deconstruction of psychoanalytic practice and theory is equally relevant (Parker & Pavón-Cuellar, 2014; Burman, 2018; Parker, 2011).

Psychoanalysis provides important contributions to the praxis of listening, particularly in placing the notion of truth on the side of the subject, which has implications for psychoanalytic practice. Consequently, the conceptions of transference and resistance become central for interpretation and critical listening.

Psychoanalytic listening implies that analysts can support transference, that is, when occupying a place of 'supposed knowledge', the psychoanalyst acts as a reference of knowledge for the subject. This refers to a position of one who supposes knowledge, working as a strategy to enable the subject to speak and to listen to their own discourse. This space provides a relationship that structures the production of the subject's knowledge, insofar as the psychoanalyst renounces domination over the encounter and, by intervening and interpreting, makes the production of effects of signification for the desiring subject possible. While subjectivity is produced in and articulated by culture, as divided subjects they are equally able to transcend the place in which they are situated and begin to assume a different relation to their desire (Rosa & Mountian, 2012).

It is through transference that psychoanalytic practice operates, that is, via the relationship between the analysand and the analyst. Two aspects are emphasised here, first, by placing the transferential relation, which also functions as an interpretative resource, to the forefront, we mobilise a distinct tool for practice. Second, the consequent need for ongoing reflexivity on the part of the analyst regarding the reproduction of power relations within the analytic setting becomes crucial, considering how gender, sexuality, race, class and age operate within and shape this relation, including the positionality of the psychoanalyst themselves. For example, Freud (1920), in the case of the Young Female Homosexual signals that the young lady would perhaps further engage with a female analyst. Ayouch and Charafeddine (2013) discuss the history and politics of homosexuality and the positioning of homosexual psychoanalysts. They underline the value of reflexivity when understanding the operation of intersectional social categories within analytic transference, which we can expand to the more general encounter between patient and health professional.

For analytic practice, transference plays a central role, such that resistance becomes another fundamental issue for practice. In this manner, resistance and transference are facets of the same phenomenon. For Freud (1912), many times resistance is egoic, occurring when patients are about to elucidate some central conflict. At that moment, free association ceases, and patients focus their attention on their relationship with the analyst. The way that resistance is interpreted is a key issue for clinical psychoanalytic practice. Here, I highlight the relevance of critical approaches to the analysand's resistance, understood as a defence mechanism, and, how in transference with the analyst, resistance is analysed through its purpose and function for the subject. Therefore, rather than simply seeking to overcome resistance, its management is incorporated into the analytic process itself. Lacan (1958/1998) further elaborates the conceptualisation of resistance switching his focus to the analyst's resistance, that is, the hindrances that occur in the one who listens rather than in the subject who speaks (Rosa & Mountian, 2012). The resistance of the analyst to listening to the subject warrants further analysis, as it can operate in ways that fix the subject in specific imaginary positions.

Taking resistance and transference into account, we can further reflect on psychoanalytic listening, which seeks to allow the subject's desire to emerge, thereby setting in motion otherwise fixed signifiers.

Rosa (1998, 1999) discusses clinical work that takes place under precarious conditions (e.g. within the context of emergency interventions, deprivation, lack of resources), wherein listening seeks to break down barriers and rescue the shared experience emerging from the encounter with the Other (Lacanian Other). For this aim, the listening must also bear witness to the subject's testimony, aimed at safeguarding memory, rather than a talk that simply repeats and updates the traumatic, which would be insufficient. For clinical listening involving socially excluded subjects, it is vital to consider the social position they occupy.

> Crucial to the specificity of clinical listening to socially excluded subjects is taking into consideration the place they occupy in the discursive logic of the [labour] market, i.e., considering the *place of leftover* that the subject occupies in the social structure and the suspension of meaning for the subject about this place in the logic of the market. This suspension of meaning is precisely what keeps them locked into a traumatic condition. The subjects' identification with this place of dejection is one of the factors that make it difficult for them to position themselves in the web of knowledge, rendering speaking impossible and marking their discourse at times, by silence. Listening to these subjects can allow them to set into motion signifying articulations that break up imaginary identifications and contribute to elucidating some of the subjective effects of the system.
>
> (Rosa & Mountian, 2012)

This type of psychoanalytic listening, therefore, does not refer to a tale told to satisfy the curiosity of the Other (Lacanian Other): neither as an exposition of suffering for the delight of the Other nor as a display of the grotesque that fixes the subject in a reified and fetishised position. *Psychoanalytic listening supposes the presence of the desiring Other in everything that it implies. Transference in this sense becomes a boundary, an organising border that mediates a potentially unrestrained jouissance.*

In line with psychoanalytic listening and practice, it is worth highlighting Castoriadis' claim regarding the end of psychoanalysis.

> The end of psychoanalysis is not 'interpretive understanding' between the analyst and the patient (which in no way is intended as such, and which is highly asymmetrical, as also is the case in pedagogy), but rather a contribution to the patient's access to his/her own autonomy (his/her capacity to challenge him/herself and lucidly to transform him/herself).
> (Castoriadis, 1991, p. 77)

Similarly, we return to the ongoing debate surrounding how to listen to the Other, offering an invitation to consider what kinds of listening are possible, as well as seeking to further understand their emancipatory possibilities. Psychoanalytic listening is focused on the subject and their desire (Freud, Lacan). Here challenges arise regarding listening to subjects who are continuously placed in the position of the Other. The process of listening, therefore, requires an ethical framework (psychoanalytic ethos) and constant reflexivity, taking into account the power relations to which the subject is submitted, without merely reducing them to a product of these, aiming rather to guarantee room for the subject's agency and desire. Similarly, Beckmann (2009) argues that through our encounter with the otherness of the Other (theirs and ours), new forms of self-understanding can emerge.

Psychoanalytic praxis allows us to deepen our understanding of the encounter between the subject and psy-practitioners. It situates the encounter as a space for ethical reflection, seeking to consider how the hindrances arising also from the resistance of the analyst can shape the therapeutic process and the inter-subjective dynamics in play. Finally, in this context, the importance of speech (voice) also arises, according to which the subject is not only the object of traditional scientific research but also actively produces it.

It is essential to consider the intersectional social categories when analysing the power relations that (re)produce the position of the Other, so as to be able to uncover the discursive rigidity of these fetishised relations. In this way, we can expand the discursive space for the subject's presence/emergence (expression), producing emancipatory possibilities and collective productions. It is through an analysis of these encounters that our ability to challenge and transform established perspectives arises, providing a platform for the emergence of the subject's voice and an acknowledgement of their own desires, agency and knowledge.

Appendix 1
Main research projects cited

Young asylum seekers, refugees and drug use early (2004–2005)

This research was produced by Early Break Young People's Drug Services Rochdale and Bury and funded by Rochdale Homelessness (Home Office), a partnership with Manchester Metropolitan University, coordinated by Ilana Mountian, supervised by Dr Khatidja Chantler and fieldwork by Bev Ebbrell (service provider). The objective of this research was to identify the needs of asylum seekers and refugees in relation to drug services (prevention and education), in order to suggest strategies for drug services in the region. The interviews were conducted with 9 asylum seekers (5 young women and 4 young men), ranging from 14 to 17 years old, and with 9 service providers (7 female and 2 male). Interviews were only recorded with service providers. Although most of the young people interviewed did not use drugs, a number of questions arose regarding drug use, refugee processes, gender and psychiatric drugs. This is groundbreaking research in this local area, as there is no available data on this specific issue. In fact, there is a lack of research that deals specifically with young asylum seekers and refugees and drug use nationwide.

Asylum-seeker experiences of access to health services: understanding the case of Manchester's Somali and Iraqi asylum seekers and refugees (2007–2008)

This research was based at the Research Institute for Health and Social Change Manchester Metropolitan University, funded by NHS – Primary Care Trust, coordinated by Judith Sixsmith and Rebecca Lawthom, conducted by Ilana Mountian and Nathan Whittle, and fieldwork together with Ryan Woolrych, and other team members. The objective of this research was to evaluate the asylum seekers' and refugees' access to health services. The study examined the experiences of asylum seekers and refugees in Manchester in relation to health beliefs, lifestyle and behaviour, to investigate their access to and inclusion in health services, and how health (and related voluntary and community) services accommodate/facilitate the access of asylum seekers and refugees. The main outcomes of this research were the acknowledgement of the cultural, social and political context of these encounters; awareness of health beliefs and lifestyle; evaluation of health services in relation to asylum seekers and refugees; and recommendations for better inclusion of these communities in health programmes.

A number of methodological strategies were applied in this participatory research, providing space for the collaboration of refugees, asylum seekers and people without legal status, in the research process. The research team met with a representative from the Chorlton Workshop who provided training opportunities for asylum seekers and refugees. Certificates were given out, and the research team provided references for research participants seeking employment. Further, attendance of refugee forums and conferences (Manchester Refugee Support Network, WAST (Women Asylum Seekers Together), WASP (Women Asylum Seekers from Pakistan, MARIM workshop)) and organisation of meetings with refugee groups and community groups were undertaken. There were more than 40 community organisations sharing information and supporting research (see appendix 2). Interpreters participated in the interviews where necessary. In-depth interviews were carried out with 14 Somali participants (8 males, 6 females) and 13 Iraqi participants (8 males, 5 females). Focus groups were held, one with asylum seekers and refugees (N-6, 4 men and 2 women) and the other with professional service providers (N-7). Health diary notes from 2 Somali men were collected.

Travestis, transsexual women and ageing (*aspectos sobre travestilidade e* envelhecimento) (2012)

This research was coordinated by Ilana Mountian and the fieldwork undertaken by Liliane Anderson, Igor Monteiro, Frederico Viana Machado, Rafaela Vasconcelos and Ilana Mountian. This study was part of the research partnership between Universidade Federal de Minas Gerais, Universidade Federal do Estado de Sao Paulo, Universidade Federal da Bahia, Universidade Federal de Pernambuco, 'The visibility of gendered bodies and their political and everyday implications' (*A visibilidade de corpos gendrados e seus desdobramentos políticos e cotidianos*), funded by CNPQ. This qualitative research sought to understand the experiences of older travesties, highlighting several important aspects concerning transphobia, human rights, health, immigration and history. Five (N-5) *travestis* were interviewed, some of whom are activists. The fieldwork was conducted by one *travesti* (activist), 2 cisgender women and 2 cisgender men.

A critical analysis of public policies on education and LGBT rights in Brazil (2013–2014)

This research, funded by the Institute of Development Studies at the University of Sussex, sought to evaluate transgender people's access to education in Brazil. It was coordinated by Ilana Mountian, supervised by Marco Aurelio Prado and Sonia Correa, and fieldwork was undertaken by Igor Monteiro and

Rodrigo Alencar. Seven (N-7) key participants from different parts of Brazil, who were either directly involved in the development of anti-homophobia policies in the education system or were researchers in this particular field, were interviewed. Interviewees included LGBT rights activists, policy makers and a trans educator. One transwoman and 6 cisgender people (male and female) were interviewed. Additionally, key documents on LGBT rights and access to education were analysed.

Intersectionality and otherness: trajectories of immigration and social networks (2015–2020)

This postdoctoral research, funded by CAPES/PNPD, was carried out at the Institute of Psychology, Universidade de Sao Paulo. The objective was to study trajectories of immigration and social networks aiming to understand how the dynamics of gender, race, class and sexuality operate in the encounter between newly arrived migrants and the hosting country. Informal interviews were carried out with migrants and service providers. During this project I participated in several forums on immigration, continued my participation in migrant health networks (since 2012), worked as a clinical supervisor for the psychosocial intervention at the Casa do Migrante and coordinated an intervention in public health in Sao Paulo (Health policy for immigrants and refugees in the city of Sao Paulo).

The public health project was developed by the Health Secretary of the City Council of Sao Paulo in partnership with PAHO/WHO (Pan American Health Organisation/World Health Organisation) in 2016 named '*Política de saúde para imigrantes e refugiados no município de Sao Paulo*' (Health policy for immigrants and refugees in the city of Sao Paulo). This project sought to combat xenophobia, racism and sexism in health services in the city of Sao Paulo (32 Public Health Units (*Unidades Básicas de Saúde* – UBS) and 5 Hospitals). Three workshops were conducted at each institution, seeking to raise awareness among health service providers and to promote a health network. The workshops were conducted by immigrants from Haiti, China, Bolivia, the Congo and Syria, among others. The meetings provided a forum for debate, information and material, including translated material for immigrants.

Otherness and immigration: intersections between gender, race and class (2012–2015)

I conducted this post-doctoral research, funded by FAPESP, at the Universidade de Sao Paulo, Brazil. The study sought to extend the debate surrounding immigrants and immigration, considering the position of the Other in discourse. It focused on Sao Paulo, particularly on newly arrived migrants. Fieldwork was undertaken at a temporary shelter for immigrants, with an ethnographic approach being adopted, undertaking visits to the shelter. I interviewed immigrants (N-10) and staff members (N-8) and coordinated a focus group with the staff.

During this research, at the *Casa do Migrante*, I worked as the clinical supervisor of the psychosocial intervention carried out by Psychology students from the University of Sao Paulo and Pontificia Universidade Católica de Sao Paulo, organised by Veredas Group (Psychoanalysis and society research group, USP) and participated in a number of immigrant forums such as the immigrant health network, Social Forum of immigration.

Drugs, gender and social imaginary (2000–2004)

My doctoral thesis undertaken at Manchester Metropolitan University and supervised by Erica Burman sought to explore discourses about drugs, gender and race. A mixed method approach was employed, including ethnography, interviews and analysis of media and advertising. The interviews and fieldwork were carried out in Brazil and Mexico, at in-patient institutions (public and private) and in informal settings and religious gatherings (Santo Daime and Mexican syncretic indigenous-Christian contexts). The interviews were conducted with drug users and health service providers (doctors and psychologists). Discourse analysis was undertaken with thirteen interviews with male and female drug users.

Appendix 2

List of community organisations assisting the research health experiences of access to health

Asylum Seekers and Refugee's Access to Health Services (2007–2008)

1. African & Caribbean Mental Health Services
2. African Community Organisation
3. African Francophone Integration Project
4. Arabic Supplementary School
5. Black HIV/AIDS Forum (BHAF)
6. Black Perspectives
7. Boaz Trust
8. British Red Cross Refugee Service (M/cr)
9. Cheetham Hill Advice Centre
10. Citizens Advice Bureau – Longsight
11. Depaul Trust – Manchester Reconnect
12. Federation of Iraqi Refugees (M/cr)
13. Greater Manchester Coalition of Disabled People
14. Greater Manchester Immigration Aid Unit
15. Haween Women's Support Group
16. Inside Track
17. Iraqi Community Welfare Association
18. Kurdish Society of Manchester
19. Manchester Asylum Seekers Team (MAST)
20. Manchester Central African Community
21. Manchester Mental Health & Social Care Trust
22. Manchester Refugee Support Network
23. MARIM
24. Medical Foundation Northwest
25. MIND
26. Mustard Tree
27. North Manchester Somali Community
28. Rainbow Group
29. RAPAR
30. Refugee Action Northwest
31. Refugee & Migrants Forum

32 Roby Outreach Project
33 Routes Project
34 Safe in the City
35 Somali Arlaadi Community
36 Somali Brava Cultural Society
37 Somali Bravanese Sisters
38 Somali Womens Group of Manchester
39 Somaliland Community Enterprise
40 The Scarman Trust Manchester
41 United Somali Bravanese
42 Whalley Range Advive and Community Resource Centre
43 Women Asylum Seekers Together (WAST)
44 Women & Children Multi-Cultural Group
45 YASP (Youth Advice & Support Project)

Bibliography

Abbing-Karahagopian, V., Huerta, C., Souverein, P. C., De Abajo, F., Leufkens, H. G. M., Slattery, J., Alvarez, Y., Miret, M., Gil, M., Oliva, B., & Hesse, U. (2014). Antidepressant prescribing in five European countries: Application of common definitions to assess the prevalence, clinical observations, and methodological implications. *European Journal of Clinical Pharmacology*, *70*, 849–857.

Acker, C. J. (1996). From all purpose anodyne to marker of deviance: Physicians' attitudes towards opiates in the US from 1890 to 1940. In R. Potter & M. Teich (Ed.), *Drugs and Narcotics in History* (pp. 114–132). Cambridge: Cambridge University Press.

Ahmed, S. (2000). *Strange Encounters – Embodied Others in Post-Colonialism*. London: Routledge.

Ahmed, S. (2003). *Affective Economies*. Seminar presented at Discourse Unit (Manchester Metropolitan University). Unpublished paper. Lancaster: Lancaster University.

Ahmed, S. (2004). Declarations of whiteness: The non-performativity of anti-racism. *Borderlands e-Journal*, *3*(2).

Ahmed, S. (2012). *On Being Included: Racism and Diversity in Institutional Life*. Durham and London: Duke University Press.

Allen, H. (1986). Psychiatry and the construction of the feminine. In P. Miller & N. Rose (Eds.), *The Power of Psychiatry* (pp. 85–111). Cambridge: Polity Press.

Alves, A. M. (2010). Envelhecimento, trajetórias e homossexualidade feminina. *Horizontes Antropológicos*, *16*(34), 213–233.

Alves, B. M., & Pitanguy, J. (1991). *O que é Feminismo*. São Paulo: Editora Brasiliense.

Amaral, M. S., Silva, T. C., Cruz, K. P., & Toneli, M. J. F. (2014). Do travestimos às travestilidades: Uma revisão do discurso acadêmico no Brasil entre 2001–2010. *Psicologia e Sociedade*, *26*(2), 301–311.

American Psychiatric Association. (1952). *Diagnostic and Statistical Manual of Mental Disorders* (1st ed.). American Psychiatric Association.

American Psychiatric Association. (1968). *Diagnostic and Statistical Manual of Mental Disorders* (2nd ed.). American Psychiatric Association.

American Psychiatric Association. (1980). *Diagnostic and Statistical Manual of Mental Disorders* (3rd ed.). American Psychiatric Association.

American Psychiatric Association. (1994). *Diagnostic and Statistical Manual of Mental Disorders* (4th ed., DSM-IV). Washington, DC: American Psychiatric Association.

American Psychiatric Association (2000). *Diagnostic and Statistical Manual of Mental Disorders* (4th ed., DSM-IV-TR). Washington, DC: American Psychiatric Association.

American Psychiatric Association. (2013). *Diagnostic and Statistical Manual of Mental Disorders* (5th ed.). American Psychiatric Association.

Anderson, S., Blok, G., & Fabian, L. (2020). *Marginalization and Space in Times of Covid-19 Lockdown Report.* Governing the Narcotic City: Hera Project.
Ansara, Y. G., & Hegarty, P. (2011). Cisgenderism in psychology: Pathologizing and misgendering children from 1999 to 2008. *Psychology & Sexuality*, *3*, 137–160.
Anthias, F., & Yuval-Davis, N. (1996). *Racialised Boundaries: Race, Nation, Gender, Colour and Class and the Anti-Racist Struggle.* London: Routledge.
Antunes, P. P. S. (2010). *Travestis envelhecem?* Dissertação de Mestrado inédita, Gerontologia da Pontifícia Universidade Católica de São Paulo.
Antunes, P. P. S., & Mercadante, E. F. (2011). Travestis, envelhecimento e velhice. *Revista Kairós Gerontologia Temática*, *14*(5), 109–132.
Anzaldúa, G. (1987). *Borderlands: The New Mestiza – La Frontera.* San Francisco: Aunt Lute Books.
Appiah, K. A. (1992). *In My Father's House: Africa in the Philosophy of Culture.* Oxford: Oxford University Press.
Apter, E. (1991). *Feminizing the Fetish: Psychoanalysis and Narrative Ob-Session in Turn-of-the-Century France.* Nova York: Cornell.
Apter, E., & Pietz, W. (Eds.). (1993). *Fetishism as Cultural Discourse.* Nova York: Cornell.
Arán, M. e Murta, D. (2009). Do diagnóstico de transtorno de identidade de gênero às redescrições da experiência da transexualidade: uma reflexão sobre gênero. *Tecnologia e saúde Physis – Revista de Saúde Coletiva*, *19*(1), 15–41.
Armas, H. (2007). *Whose Sexualities Count: Poverty Participation and Sexual Rights.* IDS Working Paper 294. Brighton: IDS.
Arnao, G. (2002). The semantics of prohibition. *Drug Text.* http://www.drugtext.org/
Ashton, H. (1991). Psychotropic-drug prescribing for women. *British Journal of Psychiatry*, *158*(Suppl. 10), 30–35.
Ayouch, T., & Charafeddine, L. B. (2013, December). A homossexualidade dos analistas: historia, política e metapsicologia. *Percurso*, *51*, 115–126.
Bacron, R. (2021). *O ativismo das mulheres sul-americanas imigrantes: um estudo de caso sobre a construção da política pública municipal em São Paulo.* Masters Dissertation. São Paulo: Programa de Pós-Graduação em Geografia Humana da Universidade de São Paulo.
Badiou, A. (2001). *Ethics: An Essay on the Understanding of Evil.* London: Verso.
Balibar, E. (2002). Is there a 'neo-racism'? In E. Balibar & I. Wallerstein (Eds.), *Race, Nation, Class: Ambiguous Identities* (pp. 17–28). London: Verso.
Balibar, E., & Wallerstein, I. (2002). *Race, Nation, Class: Ambiguous Identities.* London: Verso.
Ballestrin, L. (2013, May–August). América Latina e o giro decolonial. *Revista Brasileira de Ciência Política*, *11*, 89–117.
Bauer, G., Redman, N., Bradley, K., & Scheim, A. (2013). Sexual health of transmen who are gay, bisexual or who have sex with men: Results from Ontario, Canada. *International Journal of Transgenderism*, *14*(2), 66–74.
Beauvoir, S. (1949/1993). *The Second Sex.* London: Everyman's Library.
Beckmann, A. (2009). *The Social Construction of Sexuality and Perversion: Deconstructing Sadomasochism.* London: Palgrave Macmillan.
Benevides, B. G. (Orgs.). (2023). *Dossiê dos assassinatos e da violência contra travestis e transexuais.* São Paulo: Expressão Popular. ANTRA, IBTE.
Benevides, B. G. (2020). *Travesti ou Transsexual: tem diferença?* https://brunabenevidex.medium.com/travesti-ou-transexual-tem-diferen%C3%A7a-f8166e67e1bc
Benevides, B. G., & Nogueira, S. N. B. (Orgs.). (2021). *Dossiê dos assassinatos e da violência contra travestis e transexuais.* São Paulo: Expressão Popular, ANTRA, IBTE.

Benhabib, S., & Cornell, D. (Orgs.). (1987). *Feminismo como crítica da modernidade*. Rio de Janeiro: Rosa dos Tempos.

Berger, M. T., & Guidroz, K. (2009). *The Intersectional Approach: Transforming the Academy Through Race, Class and Gender*. Chapel Hill, NC: The University of North Carolina Press.

Berridge, V. (1989). Historical issues. In S. Mac Gregor (Ed.), *Drugs and British Society – Response to a Social Problem in the 1980s* (pp. 20–36). London: Routledge.

Berridge, V., & Edwards, G. (1987). *Opium and the People – Opiate Use in Nineteenth Century England*. London: Yale University Press and New Haven.

Bhabba, H. (1987). What does the black man want? *New Formations*, 1987 (1 Spring).

Bhabha, H. K. (1994). *The Location of Culture*. London: Routledge.

Bicev, J. T., & Aprile, M. R. (2021). Saúde E Qualidade De Vida Entre Pessoas Transexuais Do Município De São Paulo. In Centro de Estudos de Cultura Contemporânea (CEDEC) (Ed.), *Transver O Mundo: Existências e (re)existências de travestis e pessoas trans no 1° mapeamento das pessoas trans no município de São Paulo* (pp. 125–160). São Paulo: Annablume editora.

Birdwell, J., Chapman, J., & Singleton, N. (2011). *Taking Drugs Seriously: A Demos and UK Drug Commission Report on Legal Highs*. London: Demos.

Bobo, W. V., Grossardt, B. R., Lapid, M. I., Leung, J. G., Stoppel, C., Takahashi, P. Y., Hoel, R. W., Chang, Z., Lachner, C., Chauhan, M., & Flowers, L. (2019). Frequency and predictors of the potential overprescribing of antidepressants in elderly residents of a geographically defined U.S. population. *Pharmacology Research & Perspectives*, *7*, e00461.

Bourdieu, P. (1977). *Outline of a Theory of Practice*. Cambridge: Cambridge University Press.

Brah, A. (1996). *Cartographies of Diaspora: Contesting Identities*. London and New York: Routledge.

Brah, A., & Phoenix, A. (2004). Ain't I a woman? Revisiting intersectionality. *Journal of International Women's Studies*, *5*(3); Feminist Challenges: Crossing Boundaries Article 8, May.

Brasil (2015). *Secretaria Geral da Presidência da República; Secretaria Nacional de Juventude*. Brasília: Mapa do encarceramento: os jovens do Brasil.

Brasil (2019). *Ministério Da Justiça*. Infopen (Sistema De Informações Estatísticas Do Sistema Penitenciário Brasileiro).

Brauer, R., Alfageh, B., Blais, J. E., Chan, E. W., Chui, C. S. L., Hayes, J. F., Man, K. K. C., Lau, W. C. Y., Yan, V. K. C., Beykloo. M. Y., Wang, Z., Wei, L., & Wong, I. C. K. (2021). Psychotropic medicine consumption in 65 countries and regions, 2008-19: A longitudinal study. *Lancet Psychiatry*, *8*(12), 1071–1082. https://doi.org/10.1016/S2215-0366(21)00292-3

Browne, K., & Nash, C. (Eds.). (2010). *Queer Methods and Methodologies: Intersecting Queer Theories and Social Science Research*. Surrey: Ashgate.

Bucher, R. (1992). *Drogas e drogadição no Brasil*. Porto Alegre: Artes Médicas.

Burman, E. (1994). Innocents abroad: Western fantasies of childhood and the iconography of emergencies. *Disasters: The Journal of Disaster Studies and Management*, *18*(3), 238–253.

Burman, E. (1998). *Deconstructing Feminist Psychology*. London: Sage.

Burman, E. (1999). Appealing and appaling children. *Psychoanalytic Studies*, *1*(3), 285–302. London: Taylor & Francis.

Burman, E. (2000). Method, measurement and madness. In L. Holzman & J. Morss (Eds.), *Postmodern Psychologies, Societal Practice and Political Life* (pp. 49–79). London: Routledge.

Burman, E. (2003). *Discourse Analysis Means Analysing Discourse: Some Comments on Antaki, Billing, Edwards and Potter. 'Discourse Analysis Means doing Analysis: A Critique of Six Analytic Shortcomings'*. Retrieved from Discourse Analyses on Line. www.shu.ac.uk/daol/

Burman, E. (2005, October). Engendering culture in psychology. *Theory & Psychology*, *15*(4), 527–548. London: Sage Publications.

Burman, E. (2010). *Developments: Child, Image, Nation*. London: Routledge.

Burman, E. (2015). Fanon's Lacan and the traumatogenic child: Psychoanalytic reflections on the dynamics of colonialism and racism. *Theory, Culture & Society*, *33*(4), 77–101.

Burman, E. (2018). Brexit, "child as method," and the pedagogy of failure: How discourses of childhood structure the resistance of racist discourse to analysis. *Review of Education, Pedagogy, and Cultural Studies*, *40*(2), 119–143.

Burman, E., & Chantler, K. (2003). Across and between: Reflections on researching 'race', gender and mental health. *Feminism and Psychology*, *13*(3), 302–309.

Burman, E., Smailes, S., & Chantler, K. (2004, June). Culture' as a barrier to service provision and delivery: Domestic violence services for minoritized women. *Critical Social Policy, London*, *24*(3), 332–357.

Butler, J. (1993). *Bodies That Matter: On the Discursive Limits of "Sex"*. London: Routledge.

Butler, J. (1997). *Excitable Speech – A Politics of the Performative*. London: Routledge.

Butler, J. (1999). *Gender Trouble – Feminism and the Subversion of Identity*. London: Routledge.

Butler, J., Laclau, E., & Žižek, S. (2000). *Contingency, Hegemony, Universality: Contemporary Dialogues on the Left*. London: Verso.

Callaghan, J. (2015). Mothers and children? Representations of mothers in research on children's outcomes in domestic violence. *Psychology of Women Section Review*, *17*, 13–20.

Campbell, N. (2000). *Using Women – Gender, Drug Policy and Social Justice*. London: Routledge.

Carneiro, H. (2019). *Drogas: A História do Proibicionismo*. São Paulo: Autonomia Literária.

Carneiro, S. (2003). Mulheres em movimento. *Estudos avançados*, *17*(49), 117–133.

Carrijo, G. G. (2011). Imagens em trânsito: narrativas de uma travesti brasileira. In Adriana Piscitelli, Gláucia Oliveira Assis, & José Miguel Neto Olivar (Orgs.), *Gênero, sexo, amor e dinheiro: mobilidades transnacionais envolvendo o Brasil* (pp. 263–320). Campinas: UNICAMP/PAGU.

Castoriadis, C. (1991). *Philosophy, Politics, Autonomy – Essays in Political Philosophy*. Oxford: Odeon, Oxford University Press.

Castro, M. G., Abramovay, M., & Silva, L. B. (2004). *Juventudes e Sexualidade*. Brasília: UNESCO.

Cerqueira, D., & Coelho, D. S. C. (2017). *Democracia Racial E Homicídios De Jovens Negros Na Cidade Partida*. Brasília: IPEA (Instituto de Pesquisa Econômica Aplicada).

Cerqueira, D., Lima, R. S., Bueno, S., Valencia, L. I., Hanashiro, O., Machado, P. H. G., & Lima, A. S. (2017). *Atlas da violência*. Brasília: Instituto de Pesquisa Econômica Aplicada (IPEA) and Fórum Brasileiro de Segurança Pública (FBSP).

Cerqueira, D. R. D. C. C., Ferreira, H. R. S. A. C., Alves, P. P., Lima, R. S. D., Marques, D., Silva, F. A. B. D., Lunelli, I. C., Rodrigues, R. I., Lins, G. D. O. A., Armstrong, K. C., & Lira, P. (2021). *Atlas da Violência 2021*. IPEA (Instituto DE Pesquisa Econômica Aplicada). São Paulo: FBSP.

Chakrabarti, A., & Dhar, A. (2009). *Dislocation and Resettlement in Development*. Abingdon and New York: Routledge.
Chantler, K. (1998). *An Analysis of Present Drug Service Delivery to Black Communities in Greater Manchester*. Greater Manchester Drug Action Partnership and Black Drug Workers Forum North-West Publication.
Chantler, K. (2007, June). Border crossings: Nationhood, gender, culture and violence. *International Journal of Critical Psychology, 20*, 138–166.
Chantler, K., Burman, E., & Batsleer, J. (2003). South Asian women: Exploring systemic service inequalities around attempted suicide and self-harm. *European Journal of Social Work, 6*(1), 33–48. London: Taylor & Francis.
Chodorow, N. (1989). *Feminism and Psychoanalytic Theory*. New Haven, CT and London: Yale University Press.
Clements-Nolle, K., Marx, R., & Katz, M. (2006). Attempted suicide among transgender persons: The influence of gender-based discrimination and victimization. *Journal of Homosexuality, 51*(3), 53–69.
Cohen, S. (2001). *Immigration Controls, the Family and the Welfare State – A Handbook of Law, Theory, Politics and Practice for Local Authority, Voluntary Sector and Welfare State Workers and Legal Advisors*. London: Athenaeum Press.
Coll-Planas, G. (2011). La polícia del género. In M. Missé & G. Coll-Planas (Eds.), *El Género Desordenado: Críticas em torno a la patologización de la transexualidad* (pp. 55–66). Barcelona and Madrid: Egales Editorial.
Conselho Indigenista Missionário (CIMI). (2015). Report. *Violência contra os povos indígenas no Brasil*.
Cooperstock, R., & Parnell, P. (2002). Research on psychotropic drug use: A review of findings and methods. *Social Science and Medicine, 16*(12), 1179–1196.
Correa, S., Carreira, D., Simpson, K., Larrat, S., Bazzo, S., Asano, C., Galli, B., Prado, M. A. M., & Maracci, J. G. (2021). *Ofensivas Antigênero No Brasil: Políticas De Estado, Legislação, Mobilização Social*. Report. ABIA.
Costa, Pe. Gelmino A. (2011). Imigração haitiana em Manaus: Presença da Pastoral do Migrante (relato). *Travessia: Revista do Migrante, 68*, 83–88.
Courtwright, D. T. (1995). The rise and fall and rise of Cocaine in the United States. In J. Goodman, P. Lovejoy, & A. Sherratt (Eds.), *Consuming Habits – Drugs in History and Anthropology* (pp. 206–229). London: Routledge.
Craig, G. M., & O'Dell, L. (2011). Mothering on the margins: Special issue editorial. *Radical Psychology, 9*(2).
Crenitte, M. R. F. (2021). Acesso à Saúde. In C. Rebellato, M. C. A. Gomes, & M. R. F. Crenitte (Eds.), *Introdução às velhices LGBTI+* (pp. 72–78). Rio de Janeiro: Sociedade Brasileira de Geriatria e Gerontologia.
Crenshaw, K. W. (1994). Mapping the margins: Intersectionality, identity politics, and violence against women of color. In M. A. Fineman & R. Mykitiuk (Eds.), *The public nature of private violence* (pp. 93–118). New York: Routledge.
Dally, A. (1996). Anomalies and mysteries in the 'war on drugs'. In R. Potter & M. Teich (Eds.), *Drugs and Narcotics in History* (pp. 199–215). Cambridge: Cambridge University Press.
Damasceno Marizete Gouveia (2018). *Onde Se Esconde O Racismo Na Psicologia Clínica? A Experiência Da População Negra Na Invisibilidade Do Binômio Racismo e Saúde Mental*. Doctoral Thesis. Universidade de Brasilia.
Damasco, M. S., Maio, M. C., & Monteiro, S. (2012). Feminismo negro: raça, identidade e saúde reprodutiva no Brasil (1975–1993). *Revista Estudos Feministas, 20*(1), 133–151.
Danto, E. A. (2019). *As clínicas públicas de Freud: Psicanálise e Justiça Social, 1918–1938*. São Paulo: Editora Perspectiva.

Davies, J. B. (1997). *The Myth of Addiction*. Amsterdam: Harwood Academic Publishers.

Dawson, C. R. (2003). *Drug Scoping Study – Asylum Seekers and Refugee Communities*. London. Retrieved December 2004 from http://www.drugs.gov.uk/ReportsandP . . . s%20and%20refugeesfinal%20report.doc

Dean, H., & Taylor-Gooby, P. (1992). *Dependency Culture – The Explosion of a Myth*. London: Harvester Wheatsheaf.

Debert, G. G. (2010). A dissolução da vida adulta e a juventude como valor. *Horizontes Antropológicos*, *16*(34), 49–70.

De Lauretis, T. (1994). *The Practice of Love: Lesbian Sexuality and Perverse Desire*. Bloomington: Indiana University Press.

Deleuze, G., & Guattari, F. (1997). *Mil Platôs: capitalismo e esquizofrenia*. Rio de Janeiro: Editora 34.

Demaj, A. (2014). Touching race through play: Sadomasochism, phenomenology, and the intertwining of race and sexuality. *Annual Review of Critical Psychology*, *11*, 97–111.

Derrida, J. (1991). *Limited Inc*. Campinas: Papirus.

Derrida, J. (1997). *A Farmácia de Platão*. Sao Paulo: Iluminuras.

Des Jarlais, D. (1995). Harm reduction – a framework for incorporating science into drug policy. *American Journal of Public Health*, *85*(1), 10–11.

De Vos, J. (2013). *Psychologization and the Subject of Late Modernity*. New York: Palgrave Macmillan.

Dorn, N., & Lee, M. (1999). Drugs and policing in Europe: From low streets to high places. In N. South (Ed.), *Drugs – Cultures, Controls and Everyday Life* (pp. 86–102). London: Sage.

Douglas, M. (Ed.) (1987). *Constructive Drinking – Perspectives on Drink from Anthropology*. Cambridge: Cambridge University Press.

Drager, E. H., & Platero, L. (2021, November). At the margins of time and place: Transsexuals and the transvestites in trans studies. *Transgender Studies Quarterly*, *8*(4), 417–425.

Drennan, V. M., & Joseph, J. (2005). Health visiting and refugee families: Issues in professional practice. *Journal of Advanced Nursing*, *49*(2), 155–163.

Drescher, J. (2015). Out of DSM: Depathologizing homosexuality. *Behavioral Sciences (Basel, Switzerland)*, *5*(4), 565–575.

Duarte, P. D. C., Villamar, & Villarreal, M. C. (2019). Mulheres migrantes e crianças e adolescentes não acompanhados na América Latina e Caribe: algumas cifras e reflexões para o debate. In É. Sarmiento (Ed.), *E-Imigração em debate: novas abordagens na Contemporaneidade* (pp. 194–206). Rio de Janeiro: Asoec – Universo.

Dwyer, P., & Brown, D. (2005). Meeting basic needs? Forced migrants and welfare. *Social Policy and Society*, *4*(4), 369–380. Cambridge: Cambridge University Press.

Engel, M. (1997). Psiquiatria e Feminilidade. In M. Del Priore (Ed.), *História das Mulheres no Brasil* (pp. 322–361). Sao Paulo: Editora Contexto.

Escohotado, A. (1998). *Historia de las drogas* (Vols. 1, 2 and 3). Madrid: Allianza Editorial.

Ettorre, B. (1989). Women, substance abuse and self-help. In S. MacGregor (Ed.), *Drugs and British Society – Responses to a Social Problem in the Eighties* (pp. 101–115). London: Routledge.

Ettorre, E. (1992). *Women and Substance Use*. London: Macmillan.

Ettorre, E. (Ed.). (2005). *Making Lesbians Visible in the Substance Use Field*. New York: Harrington Park Press.

Ettorre, E., & Riska, E. (1995). *Gendered Moods – Psychotropics and Society*. London: Routledge.

Eze, E. (Ed.). (1997). *Race and the Enlightenment: A Reader*. Cambridge, MA: Blackwell.

Facchini, R. (2009). Entre compassos e descompassos: um olhar para o "campo" e para a "arena" do movimento LGBT brasileiro. *Bagoas*, *4*, 131–158.

Facchini, R., Carmo, Í. N., & Lima, S. P. (2020). Movimentos feminista, negro e LGBTI no Brasil: sujeitos, teias e enquadramentos. *Educação & Sociedade*, *41*, 1–22.

Fairclough, N. (1992). *Discourse and Social Change*. Cambridge: Polity Press.

Fairclough, N. (1995). *Critical Discourse Analysis: The Critical Study of Language*. London: Longman.

Fang, M. L., Sixsmith, J., Lawthom, R., Mountian, I., & Shahrin, A. (2015). Experiencing 'pathologized presence and normalized absence'; understanding health related experiences and access to health care among Iraqi and Somali asylum seekers, refugees and persons without legal status. *BMC Public Health*, *15*, 923.

Fanon, F. (1986). *Black Skin, White Masks*. London: Pluto.

Fassin, D., & Rechtman, R. (2009). *The Empire of Trauma: An Inquiry into the Condition of Victimhood*. Princeton and Oxford: Princeton University Press.

Fausto, B. (1996). *História do Brasil*. Sao Paulo: EDUSP.

Feaster, F., & Wood, B. (2004). *The Golden Age of Exploitation*, interviewed by Johnson, G. http://imagesjournal.com/issue08/features/exploitation/

Federici, S. (1975). *Wages Against Housework*. Bristol: Falling Wall Press Ltd.

Federici, S. (2017). *Calibã e a Bruxa: mulheres, corpo e acumulação primitiva*. Tradução Coletivo Sycorax. São Paulo: Editora Elefante.

Feldman, R. (2006). Primary health care for refugees and asylum seekers: A review of the literature and a framework for services. *Public Health*, *120*(9), 809–816.

Fell, P., & Hayes, D. (2007). *What Are They Doing Here? A Critical Guide to Asylum and Immigration*. Birmingham: Venture Press.

Fernandes, D., & Baeninger, R. (Org.). (2020). *Impactos da Pandemia de Covid-19 nas Migrações Internacionais no Brasil. Resultados De Pesquisa*. PUC/Minas, UNICAMP.

Fernandes, J., Barroso, K. A. A., & Pocahy, F. (2015). Gênero, sexualidade e envelhecimento: uma revisão sistemática da literatura. *Clínica & Cultura*, *4*(1), 14–28.

Fernandes, J. A. (2011). *Selvagens Bebedeiras: Álcool, Embriaguez e Contatos Culturais no Brasil Colonia (XVI–XVII)*. São Paulo: Alameda Casa Editorial.

Fernando, S. (1988). *Race and Culture in Psychiatry*. London and New York: Routledge.

Fernando, S. (2012, June). Race and culture issues in mental health and some thoughts on ethnic identity. *Counselling Psychology Quarterly*, *25*(2), 113–123.

Figueiredo, R., & Cavallari, C. (Eds.). (2020, December). Boletim do Instituto da Saúde. *Drogas & 30 Anos de Redução de Danos*, *21*(2).

Finkelstein, N. (1996). Using the relational model as a context for treating pregnant and parenting chemically dependent women. In B. Underhill & D. Finnegan (Eds.), *Chemical Dependency – Women at Risk* (pp. 23–44). London: Harrington Press.

Fiocruz (2020). https://mooc.campusvirtual.fiocruz.br/rea/covid-prisional/unidade1.html

Foucault, M. (1973). *The Birth of the Clinic: An Archaeology of Medical Perception*. London: Routledge.

Foucault, M. (1974/2012). *O Poder Psiquiátrico*. São Paulo: Martins Fontes.

Foucault, M. (1976/2007). *História da Sexualidade*. Rio de Janeiro: Graal.

Foucault, M. (1978). *The History of Sexuality, Volume 1: An Introduction*. New York: Random House.

Foucault, M. (1991). *Discipline and Punishment – The Birth of the Prison*. London: Penguin Books.

Foucault, M. (1998). *The Will to Knowledge – The History of Sexuality I*. London: Penguin Books.

Foucault, M. (2006). *History of Madness*. London: Routledge.

Foucault, M. (2010). *The Archeology of Knowledge*. London: Routledge.

Franks, W., Gawn, N., & Bowden, G. (2007). Barriers to access to mental health services for migrant workers, refugees and asylum seekers. Journal of Public Mental Health, 6(1), 33–41.
Freitas, P. (2013). Bolivianos(as) por entre oficinas de costura na cidade de São Paulo: novos aspectos da dinâmica migratória no século 21. In R. Baeninger (Ed.), *Migrações Internacionais*. Coleção Por Dentro do Estado de São Paulo (vol. 9, p. 77–102). Campinas: Núcleo de Estudos da população.
Freud, S. (1912/1976). Recomendações aos médicos que exercem a psicanálise. *Obras Completas. Rio de Janeiro: Imago* (Vol. XII, pp. 145–159). Edição Standard Brasileira.
Freud, S. (1913/1976). Sobre o início do tratamento (Novas recomendações sobre a técnica da psicanálise I). *Obras Completas. Rio de Janeiro: Imago* (Vol. XII, pp. 161–187). Edição Standard Brasileira.
Freud, S. (1918). Lines of advance in psychoanalytic psychotherapy. *Standard Edition, 17*, 157–168.
Freud, S. (1920/1955). The psychogenesis of a case of homosexuality in a woman. In *The Standard Edition of the Complete Psychological Works of Sigmund Freud* (Vol. XVIII, pp. 145–172). London: Hogarth Press.
Freud, S. (1921). *Group Psychology and the Analysis of the Ego*. The Standard Edition of the Complete Psychological Works of Sigmund Freud.
Freud, S. (1977a). Fetishism. In A. Richards (Ed.), *On Sexuality – Three Essays on the Theory of Sexuality and Other Works* (pp. 345–357). London: Penguin Books.
Freud, S. (1977b). *On Sexuality – Three Essays on the Theory of Sexuality and Other Works*. London: Penguin Books.
Freyre, G. (1946). *The Masters and the Slaves: A Study in the Development of Brazilian Civilization*. New York: Knopf.
Frosh, S. (1995). Time, space and otherness. In S. Pile & N. Thrift (Eds.), *Mapping the Subject – Geographies of Cultural Transformation* (pp. 291–308). London: Routledge.
Frosh, S. (1999). *The Politics of Psychoanalysis: An Introduction to Freudian and Post-Freudian Theory*. New York: New York University Press.
Frosh, S. (2005). *Hate and the 'Jewish Science': Anti-Semitism, Nazism and Psychoanalysis*. New York: Palgrave Macmillan.
Frosh, S. (2014). Desintegrating narrative research with Lacan. In I. Parker & D. Pavón-Cuellar (Eds.), *Lacan, Discourse, Event: New Psychoanalytic Approaches to Textual Indeterminacy* (pp. 17–26). London: Routledge.
Galvão, J. (2002). 1980–2001 – *Uma Cronologia da Epidemia de HIV/AIDS no Brasil e no Mundo*. Rio de Janeiro: ABIA.
Gamman, L., & Makinen, M. (1994). *Female Fetishism: A New Look*. London: Lawrence and Wishart.
Ghatak, S. (2010). "The opium wars": The biopolitics of narcotic control in the United States, 1914–1935. *Critical Criminology, 18*, 41–56.
Ghebrehewet, S., Regan, M., Benons, L., & Knowles, J. (2002). Provision of services to asylum seekers. Are there lessons from the experience with Kosovan refugees? *Journal of Epidemiology Community Health, 56*, 223–226.
Giacco, D., & Priebe, S. (2018). Mental health care for adult refugees in high-income countries. *Epidemiology and Psychiatric Sciences, 27*(2), 109–116.
Giami, A. (2015). Between DSM and ICD: Paraphilias and the transformation of sexual norms. *Archives of Sexual Behavior, 44*, 1127–1138.
Gianesi, A. P. L., & Mountian, I. (2019, July–December). Psicanálise e política: debates feministas para a psicanálise. *Clínica & Cultura, 8*(2), 2–20.
Gibson, N., & Beneduce, R. (2019). *Introduction to Frantz Fanon, Psychiatry and Politics*. Washington, DC: Rowman & Littlefield Publishers.

Gilroy, P. (2000). *Between Camps: Race, Identity and Nationalism at the End of the Colour Line*. London: Penguin Press.
Giordano, C. (2011). Translating Fanon in the Italian context: Rethinking the ethics of treatment in psychiatry. *Transcultural Psychiatry*, *48*(3), 228–256.
Goldberg, T. (1999). *Demystifying Drugs – A Psychosocial Perspective*. London: Macmillan Press.
Gonzalez, L. (1984). Racismo e sexismo na cultura brasileira. In *Revista Ciências Sociais Hoje* (pp. 223–244). ANPOCS.
Gonzalez, L. (2020). *Por um feminismo Afro Latino Americano*. São Paulo: Zahar.
Goodman, J., Lovejoy, P., & Sherratt, A. (1995). *Consuming Habits – Drugs in History and Anthropology*. London: Routledge.
Gordo-López, A. (2002). El estado actual de la psicología crítica. *Atenea Digital*, *1*.
Gordon, L. R. (2006/Summer 2005). Through the zone of nonbeing: A reading of *Black Skin, White Masks* in celebration of Fanon's eightieth birthday. *The C.L.R. James Journal*, *11*(1), 1–43.
Gordon, L. R. (2007, Summer). Through the Hellish zone of nonbeing: Thinking through Fanon, disaster, and the damned of the earth. *Human Architecture: Journal of the Sociology of Self-Knowledge*, *5*, 5–12.
Graham, L., Crissman, H., Tocco, J., Hughes, L., Snow, R., & Padilla, M. (2014). Interpersonal relationships and social support in transitioning narratives of black transgender women in Detroit. *International Journal of Transgenderism*, *15*(2), 100–113.
Grech, S. (2011, February). Recolonising debates or perpetuated coloniality? Decentring the spaces of disability, development and community in the global South. *International Journal of Inclusive Education*, *15*(1), 87–100.
Grech, S. (2015). Decolonising eurocentric disability studies: Why colonialism matters in the disability and global South debate. *Social Identities*, *21*(1), 6–21.
Grosz, E. (1995). *Space, Time and Perversion: Essays on the Politics of Bodies*. London: Routledge.
Grupo Gay da Bahia (GGB) (2021). *Mortes Violentas De LGBT+ No Brasil*. Report.
Gurfinkel, D. (1996). A Droga e a Coisa: Sobre a Delimitação do Conceito de Toxicomania. In C. Cohen, F. C. Ferraz, & M. Segre (Eds.), *Saúde Mental, Crime e Justiça* (pp. 225–238). Sao Paulo: Edusp.
Gusfield, J. (1987). Passage to play: Rituals of drinking time in American Society. In M. Douglas (Ed.), *Constructive Drinking – Perspectives on Drink from Anthropology*. Cambridge: Cambridge University Press.
Gusfield, J. (1997). The culture of public problems: Drinking-driving and the symbolic order. In A. M. Brandt & P. Rozin (Ed.), *Morality and Health* (pp. 201–229). London: Routledge.
Haaken, J. (2002). Bitch and fem psychology: Women, aggression and psychoanalytic social theory. *Journal for the Psychoanalysis of Culture and Society*, *7*(2), 202–215.
Hacking, I. (2006). Kinds of people: Moving targets. *Proceedings of the British Academy*, *151*, 285–318.
Halberstam, J. (2011). *The Queer Art of Failure*. Durham, NC: Duke University Press.
Hall, S. (2008). *Da Diáspora: Identidades e Mediações Culturais*. Belo Horizonte: Editora UFMG.
Haraway, D. (1988). Situated knowledges: The science question in feminism and the privilege of partial perspective. *Feminist Studies*, *14*(3), 575–599.
Haraway, D. J. (1991). *Simians, Cyborgs, and Women: The Reinvention of Nature*. London: Free Association Books.
Harding, S. (1986). Is there a feminist method? In S. Harding (Ed.), *Feminism and Methodology* (pp. 1–14). Buckingham: Open University Press.

Harding, S. (1996). Rethinking standpoint epistemology: What is 'strong objectivity'? In E. F. Keller & H. Longino (Eds.), *Feminism and Science – Oxford Readings in Feminism* (pp. 235–248). Oxford: Oxford Press.

Harradine, A. (2004). *A City Perspective on EU Asylum, Immigration and Integration Policies*. Public Consultation on the Future Guidelines for the New Programme on Establishment of an Area of Freedom, Security and Justice. Response from the Greater London Authority, Brussels. www.europelandofasylum.net

Harris, J., & Roberts, K. (2004). 'Not our problem': The provision of services to disabled refugees and asylum seekers. In D. Hayes & B. Humphries (Eds.), *Social Work, Immigration and Asylum – Debates, Dilemmas and Ethical Issues for Social Work and Social Care Practice* (pp. 151–161). London: Jessica Kingsley Publishers.

Harrison, B. (1971). *Drink and the Victorians – The Temperance Question in England 1815–1972*. London: Faber and Faber.

Hayes, D. (2004). History and context: The impact of immigration control on welfare delivery. In D. Hayes & B. Humphries (Eds.), *Social Work, Immigration and Asylum – Debates, Dilemmas and Ethical Issues for Social Work and Social Care Practice* (pp. 11–29). London: Jessica Kingsley Publishers.

Healy, D. (2004). *Let Them Eat Prozac – The Unhealthy Relationship Between the Pharmaceutical Industry and Depression*. New York: New York University Press.

Hegarty, P. (2007). From genius inverts to gendered intelligence: Lewis Terman and the power of the norm. *History of Psychology*, *10*(2), 132–155.

Heidegger, M. (1997). *Being and Time*. Oxford: Blackwell.

Henderson, S. (1999). Drugs and culture: The question of gender. In N. South (Ed.), *Drugs – Cultures, Controls and Everyday Life* (pp. 36–48). London: Sage.

Henriques, J., Hollway, W., Urwin, C., Venn, C., Walkerdine, V. (1984). *Changing the Subject: Psychology, Social Regulation and Subjectivity*. London: Methuen.

Herzberg, D. L. (2009). *Happy Pills in America – from Miltown to Prozac*. Baltimore, MD: John Hopkins University Press.

Hickling, F. W. (2020, February). Owning our madness: Contributions of Jamaican psychiatry to decolonizing Global Mental Health. *Transcultural Psychiatry*, *57*(1), 19–31.

Hickman, Timothy A. (2000). Drugs and race in American culture: Orientalism in the turn-of-the-century discourse of narcotic addiction. *American Studies*, *41*(1), 71–91.

Hill, C., Bilge, S., & Bilge, S. (2016). *Intersectionality (Key Concepts)*. Cambridge: Polity Press.

Hill Collins, P. (2000). *Black Feminist Thought: Knowledge, Consciousness, and the Politics of Empowerment* (2nd ed.). London: Routledge.

Hockey, J. (1993). Women and health. In D. Richardson & V. Robinson (Eds.), *Introducing Women's Studies* (pp. 250–271). London: Macmillan.

Hollanda, H. B. (Ed.). (2019). *Pensamento Feminista Brasileiro: formação e contexto*. Rio de Janeiro: Bazar do Tempo.

Hollingworth, L. S. (1914). Variability as related to sex differences in achievement: A critique. *American Journal of Sociology*, *19*, 510–530.

Home Department (1999). *The Stephen Lawrence Inquiry: Report of an Inquiry by Sir William Macpherson of Cluny*. London: Stationery Office.

Hook, D. (Ed.). (2004). *Critical Psychology*. Lansdowne: UCT Press.

Hook, D. (2005). A critical psychology of the post-colonial. *Theory and Psychology*, *15*(4), 475–503.

Hook, D. (2012). *A Critical Psychology of the Postcolonial: The Mind of Apartheid*. London: Routledge.

hooks, b. (1984/2005). Black women: Shaping feminist theory. In A. Cudd & R. O. Andreasen (Eds.), *Feminist Theory: A Philosophical Anthology*. Oxford: Blackwell.

Hunt, N., & Stevens, A. (2004). Whose harm? Harm reduction and the shift to coercion in UK drug policy. *Social Policy & Society*, *3*(4), 333–342.

Hutta, J. S., & Balzer, C. (2013). Identidades e cidadania em construção: historização do 'T' nas políticas de antiviolência LGBT no Brasil. In J. M. Silva, M. J. Ornat, & A. B. Chimin, Jr. (Org.), *Geografias malditas: corpos, sexualidades e espaços* (pp. 311–338). Ponta Grossa: Todapalavra.

Illich, I. (1995). *Limits to Medicine – Medical Nemesis: The Exploration of Health*. London: Marion Boyars.

Inciardi, J., & Harrison, L. (2000). *Harm Reduction: National and International Perspectives*. London: Sage.

Instituto Brasileiro de Ciências Criminais (IBCCRIM) (2011). *Número de mulheres encarceladas cresceu nos últimos 5 anos*. https://www.ibccrim.org.br/noticia/13838-Nmero-de-mulheres-encarceradas-cresceu-nos-ltimos-5-anos

Instituto Brasileiro de Geografia e Estatística (IBGE) (2012). *Síntese de Indicadores Sociais: Uma Análise das Condições de Vida da População Brasileira*. Rio de Janeiro: IBGE.

Instituto de Pesquisa Econômica Aplicada (IPEA) (2013). *Duas Décadas de Desigualdade e Pobreza no Brasil Medidas Pela PNAD/IBGE*. Report No. 159. Brasília: IPEA.

Instituto de Pesquisa Econômica Aplicada (IPEA) (2021). *Atlas da Violência*. Brasília: IPEA.

Instituto Terra, Trabalho e Cidadania (ITTC) (2015). *Infográfico mulheres e tráfico de drogas: Um sentença tripla*. Infográficos. http://ittc.org.br/infografico-mulheres-e-trafico-de-drogas-uma-sentenca-tripla/

Irineu, B. A., & Froemming, C. N. (2012, July). Homofobia, Sexismo e Educação: Notas Sobre as Possibilidades de Enfrentamento a Violência a Partir de um Projeto de Extensão Universitária. *Universidade do Estado do Rio de Janeiro: Revista Advir*, 75–90.

Jacobson, B. (1981). *The Lady Killers – Why Smoking Is a Feminist Issue*. London: Pluto Press.

Junqueira, R. D. (Org.). (2009). *Diversidade Sexual na Educação: problematizações sobre a homofobia nas escolas*. Brasília: Secretaria de Educação Continuada, Alfabetização e Diversidade (Secad/MEC) e Organização das Nações Unidas para a Educação, a Ciência e a Cultura (UNESCO).

Karam, M. L. (2007). Legislações proibicionistas em matéria de drogas e danos aos direitos fundamentais. *Verve*, *12*, 181–212.

Karam, M. L. (2008). A lei 11.343/06 e os repetidos danos do proibicionismo. In B. C. Labate, S. Goulart, M. Fiore, E. MacRae, & H. Carneiro (org.), *Drogas e cultura: novas perspectivas* (pp. 105–122). Salvador: EDUFBA.

Katz, S. (1997). Secular morality. In A. Brandt & P. Rozin (Eds.), *Morality and Health* (pp. 297–330). London: Routledge.

Keane, H. (1999). Adventures of the addicted brain. *Australian Feminist Studies*, *14*(29), 63–76.

Keire, M. L. (1998). Dope fiends and degenerates: The gendering of addiction in the early twentieth century. *Journal of Social History*, *31*(4), 809–822.

Keller, E. F. (1996). Feminism and science. In E. F. Keller & H. E. Longino (Eds.), *Feminism and Science* (pp. 28–40). Oxford: Oxford University Press.

Keller, E. F., & Longino, H. (Eds.). (1996). *Feminism and Science – Oxford Readings in Feminism*. Oxford: Oxford Press.

Kilomba, G. (2019). *Memórias da Plantação: Episódios de Racismo Cotidiano*. Rio de Janeiro: Cobogó.

Kimmel, D. (2014). Lesbian, gay, bisexual, and transgender aging concerns. *Clinical Gerontologist*, *37*, 49–63.

Klee, H., Jackson, M., & Lewis, S. (Eds.). (2002). *Drug Misuse and Motherhood*. London: Routledge.

Kohn, M. (1992). *Dope Girls: The Birth of the British Underground*. London: Lawrence and Wishart.

Krafft-Ebing, R. (1895). *Psychopathia Sexualis with Special Reference to Contrary Sexual Instinct. A Medico-Legal Study*. London: F.A. Davis Company.

Krenak, A. (2020). *O Amanhã não está à Venda*. São Paulo: Companhia das Letras.

Kulick, D. (1998). *Travesti: Sex, Gender, and Culture Among Brazilian Transgendered Prostitutes*. Chicago: University of Chicago.

Lacan, J. (1958/1998). A direção do tratamento e os princípios de seu poder. In *Escritos*. Rio de Janeiro: Jorge Zahar.

Lacan, J. (1989). *Écrits – A Selection*. London: Tavistock/Routledge.

Lacan, J. (1991). The seminar of Jacques Lacan. In J.-A. Miller (Ed.), *Book I – Freud's Papers on Techniques – 1953–1954*. London: W.W. Norton & Company.

Lacan, J. (1992). The seminar of Jacques Lacan. In J.-A. Miller (Ed.), *The Ethics of Psychoanalysis (1959–1960)*. London: Routledge.

Lacan, J. (1994). *Four Fundamental Concepts of Psycho-Analysis*. London: Penguin.

Lacan, J. (1995). *A Relação de Objeto – Livro 4*. Rio de Janeiro: Jorge Zahar Editor.

Laqueur, T. (1990). *Making Sex: Body and Gender from the Greeks to Freud*. Cambridge: Harvard University Press.

Lau, L. S., & Rodgers, G. (2021). Cultural competence in refugee service settings: A scoping review. *Health Equity*, *5*(1), 124–134. https://doi.org/10.1089/heq.2020.0094

Layton, L., Hollander, N. C., & Gutwill, S. (Eds.). (2006). *Psychoanalysis, Class and Politics: Encounters in the Clinical Setting*. New York: Routledge.

Lemgruber, J., Telles, A. C., Neder, R., Borges, D., Vargas, K., & Siracusa, M. (2021). *Um Tiro no Pé: Impactos da proibição das drogas no orçamento do sistema de justiça criminal do Rio de Janeiro e São Paulo*. Rio de Janeiro: Centro de estudos de segurança e cidadania.

Littlewood, R. (1994). Symptoms, struggles and functions: What does the overdose represent? In M. McDonald (Ed.), *Gender, Drink and Drugs* (pp. 79–97). Oxford: Berg.

Littlewood, R., & Lipsedge, M. (1989). *Aliens and Alienists – Ethnic Minorities and Psychiatry*. London: Unwin Hyman Ltd.

Loose, R. (2002a). *The Subject of Addiction – Psychoanalysis and the Administration of Enjoyment*. London: Karnak.

Loose, R. (2002b). A Lacanian approach to clinical diagnosis and addiction. In J. Glynos & Y. Stavrakakis (Eds.), *Lacan and Science* (pp. 263–289). London: Karnak.

Lopes, R. G. C. (1999). *As Interpretações Sociais da Saúde na Velhice, Refletidas no Uso do Medicamento*. Doctorate Research, Faculty of Health Care Studies, University de São Paulo.

Lorde, A. (1980/1997). Age, race, class and sex – Women redefining difference. In A. McClintock, A. Mufti, & E. Shohat (Eds.), *Dangerous Liaisons: Gender, Nation and Postcolonial Perspectives* (pp. 374–380). Minneapolis: Minnesota University Press.

Lorde, A. (1984/2007). The master's tools will never dismantle the master's house. In *Sister Outsider: Essays and Speeches* (pp. 110–114). Berkeley: Crossing Press.

Lunbeck, E. (1994). *The Psychiatric Persuasion – Knowledge, Gender and Power in Modern America*. Princeton, NJ: Princeton University Press.

Macedo, F., Machado, P. S., & Mountian, I. (2021). O cuidado com gestantes que usam drogas: análise de práticas em políticas públicas de saúde no Sul do Brasil. *Physis Revista de Saúde Coletiva*, *31*, e310223.

Macey, D. (1994). Introduction. In J. Lacan (Ed.), *Four Fundamental Concepts of Psycho-Analysis*. London: Penguin.

Machado, A. R., & Miranda, P. S. C. (2007). Fragmentos da história da atenção à saúde para usuários de álcool e outras drogas no Brasil: da Justiça à Saúde Pública. *História, Ciências, Saúde –Manguinhos*, *14*(3), 801–821.

Machado, F. V., Barnat, F., & Mattos, R. (Eds.). (2017). *A Diversidade e a Livre Expressão Sexual entre as Ruas, as Redes e as Políticas Públicas*. Porto Alegre: Editora Unida.

MacRae, E. (1998). Santo Daime and Santa Maria – The licit ritual use of ayahuasca and the illicit use of Cannabis in a Brazilian Amazonian Religion. *International Drug of Drug Policy*, *9*, 325–338.

MacRae, E. (2016a). Canabis, Racismo, Resistência, Cultura e Espiritualidade. In E. MacRae & W. C. Alves (Eds.), *Fumo de Angola: Canabis, Racismo, Resistência, Cultura e Espiritualidade* (pp. 25–58). Salvador: EDUFBA.

MacRae, E. (2016b). Santo Daime e Santa Maria: usos religiosos de substâncias psicoativas lícitas e ilícitas. In E. MacRae & W. C. Alves (Eds.), *Fumo de Angola: Canabis, Racismo, Resistência, Cultura e Espiritualidade* (pp. 445–472). Salvador: EDUFBA.

MacRae, E., & Alves, W. C. (Eds.). (2016). *Fumo de Angola: Canabis, Racismo, Resistência, Cultura e Espiritualidade*. Salvador: EDUFBA.

MacRae, E., & Simões, J. A. (2004). *Rodas de fumo: o uso da maconha entre camadas médias urbanas*. Salvador: EDUFBA.

Madeira, L. M., Furtado, B. A., & Dill, A. R. (2021). *Vida: simulando violência doméstica em tempos de quarentena*. Brasília: IPEA (Instituto De Pesquisa Econômica Aplicada).

Maito, D. C., Panuncio-Pinto, M. P., & Vieira, E. M. (2021). Violence against women at the university: Sexual violence highlighted. *Journal of Sexual Medicine*, *5*(1), 1068.

Malheiro, L. (2020). *Tornar-se Mulher Usuária de Crack: cultura e política sobre drogas*. Rio de Janeiro: Editora Telha.

Malone, K. (2006). Regulations and standards for psychoanalysis: The place of the other in psychoanalysis and its teaching. *European Journal of Psychotherapy and Counseling*, *8*, 269–284.

Marconi, A. M., Myers, U. S., Hanson, B., Nolan, S., & Sarrouf, E. B. (2023). Psychiatric medication prescriptions increasing for college students above and beyond the COVID-19 pandemic. *Scientific Reports*, *13*(1), 19063. https://doi.org/10.1038/s41598-023-46303-9

Margo, G. (2016). *The Social Imaginary on Women Who Use Drugs: Decoding Contemporary Drug Discourses in the Russian Federation*. Master's Dissertation, Central European University, Critical Gender Studies.

Martinez-Guzman, A., Montenegro, M., & Pujol, J. (2014). Towards a situated approach to sex/gender identities. *Annual Review of Critical Psychology*, *11*, 5–21.

Marx, K. (1990). *Capital* (Vol. 1). London: Penguin Books.

Masur, J., & Carlini, E. L. (1994). *Drogas – Subsídios para uma discussão*. Sao Paulo: Editora Brasiliense.

Mathon, B., Amelot, A., Clemenceau, S., Carpentier, A., & Boch, A. (2018, June). Commentary: La Pitié-Salpêtrière hospital in Paris: The historic cradle of neurosurgery. *Neurosurgery*, *82*(6), 164–174.

Mayor of London (2004a). *Destitution by Design – Withdrawal of Support from in-Country Asylum Applications: An Impact Assessment for London*. London: Greater London Authority.

Mayor of London (2004b). *Offering More Than They Borrow – Refugee Children in London*. London: Greater London Authority.

Mazzon, J. A. (2009). *Projeto de Estudo Sobre Ações Discriminatórias no Âmbito Escolar, Organizadas de Acordo com Áreas Temáticas, a Saber, Étnico-racial, Gênero, Geracional, Territorial, Necessidades Especiais, Socioeconômica e Orientação Sexual*. Ministério da Educação, Instituto nacional de estudos e pesquisas educacionais (INEP).

Mbembe, A. (2020). *O Direito Universal à Respiração*. São Paulo: Editora N-1.

Mbembe, M. (2001). As Formas Africanas de Auto-Inscrição. *Estudos Afro-Asiáticos*, *23*(1), 171–209.
McClintock, A. (1995). *Imperial Leather – Race, Gender and Sexuality in the Colonial Contest*. London: Routledge.
McColl, H., & Johnson, S. (2006). Characteristics and needs of asylum seekers and refugees in contact with London community mental health teams – A descriptive investigation. *Social Psychiatry and Psychiatric Epidemiology*, *41*(10), 789–795.
McDonald, M. (1994). *Gender, Drink and Drugs*. Oxford: Berg.
McKenna, T. (1992). *Food of the Gods – The Search for the Original Tree of Knowledge. A Radical History of Plants, Drugs and Human Evolution*. London: Rider Publications.
McMaster, D. (2003). Asylum seekers and the politics of citizenship. *Borderlands e-journal*, *2*(1).
McMurran, M. (1994). *The Psychology of Addiction*. London: Taylor & Francis.
McRuer, R. (2011). Disabling sex: Notes for a crip theory of sexuality. *GLQ: Journal of Lesbian and Gay Studies*, *17*(1), 107–117.
McSweeney, T., Stevens, A., Hunt, N., & Turnbull, P. (2006). Twisting arms or a helping hand? Assessing the impact of 'coerced' and comparable 'voluntary' drug treatment options. *British Journal of Criminology*, 1–21.
McSweeney, T., Turnbull, P. J., & Hough, M. (2008). *Tackling Drug Markets and Distribution Networks in the UK – A Review of the Recent Literature*. Institute for Criminal Policy Research. London: UK Drug Policy Commission.
Mello, L., Brito, W., & Maroja, D. (2012). Políticas Públicas Para a População LGBT no Brasil: Notas Sobre Alcances e Possibilidades. *Cadernos Pagu*, *39*, 403–429.
Mello, L., Freitas, F., Pedrosa, C. B., & Brito, W. (2010). Para Além de um Kit Anti-homofobia: Políticas Públicas de Educação Para a População LGBT no Brasil. *Bagoas: Estudos Gays gêneros e sexualidades*, 7, 99–123.
Metzl, J. (2010). *The Protest Psychosis: How Schizophrenia Became a Black Disease*. Boston, MA: Beacon Press.
Michaels, W. B. (1992). Race into culture: A critical genealogy of cultural identity. *Critical Inquiry*, *18*(4), 655–685.
Mignolo, W. D. (2007). Introduction: Coloniality of power and de-colonial thinking. *Cultural Studies*, *21*(2–3), 155–167.
Mills, C. (2014). *Decolonising Global Mental Health: The Psychiatrisation of the Majority World*. London: Routledge.
Ministério da Justiça (2016). Departamento Penitenciário Nacional. In *Levantamento nacional de informação penitenciárias*. Brasília: INFOPEN Mulheres. http://www.justica.gov.br/noticias/estudo-traca-perfil-da-populacao-penitenciaria-feminina-no-brasil/relatorio-infopen-mulheres.pdf
Missé, M., & Coll-Planas, G. (Org.). (2011). *El género desordenado: críticas en torno de la patologización de la transexualidad*. Barcelona-Madrid: Egales Editorial.
Mitropoulos, A. (2008). The materialisation of race in multiculture. In *Race/Matter – Materialism and the Politics of Racialization*. http://www.darkmatter101.org/site/2008/02/23/the-materialisation-of-race-in-multiculture/
Mohanty, C. T. (1994). Under western eyes: Feminist scholarship and colonial discourses. In P. Williams & L. Chrisman (Eds.), *Colonial Discourse and Post-Colonial Theory: A Reader* (pp. 196–220). New York: Columbia University Press.
Moi, T. (1985). *Sexual/Textual Politics*. London: Methuen. Quoted in Frosh, Stephen (1995). Time, space and otherness. In S. Pile & N. Thrift (Eds.), *Mapping the Subject – Geographies of Cultural Transformation* (pp. 291–308). London: Routledge.
Moleiro, C., & Pinto, N. (2015). Sexual orientation and gender identity: Review of concepts, controversies and their relation to psychopathology classification systems. *Frontiers in Psychology*, *6*, 1511.

Moncrieff, J. (2008). The creation of the concept of an antidepressant: An historical analysis. *Social Science & Medicine*, *66*, 2346–2355.
Moncrieff, J. (2010). Psychiatric diagnosis as a political device. *Social Theory & Health*, *8*, 370–382.
Moore, M., Yuen, H. M., Dunn, N., Mullee, M. A., Maskell, J., & Kendrick, T. (2009). Explaining the rise in antidepressant prescribing: A descriptive study using the general practice research database. *British Medical Journal*, *339*, 1–7.
Morgan, G., Melluish, S., & Welham, A. (2017, November). Exploring the relationship between postmigratory stressors and mental health for asylum seekers and refused asylum seekers in the UK. *Transcultural Psychiatry*, *54*, 653–674.
Motta, A. B. (2004). Gênero, idades e gerações. *Caderno CRH*, *17*(42), 349–355.
Mouffe, C. (1998, Summer). The radical centre: A politics without adversary. *Soundings*, *9*, 11–23.
Mountian, A. G., & Diaz, M. D. M. (2020). Effects of retirement on the health of elderly people in São Paulo, Brazil. *Applied Economics*, *52*(28), 2991–3003.
Mountian, I. (2005). Images of women and drugs. In B. Biglia, J. Clark, J. Motzkau, & A. Zavos (Eds.), *Feminisms and Activisms. Annual Review of Critical Psychology*, *4*, 81–95. Discourse Unit: Manchester.
Mountian, I. (2007). Mujeres bajo Control. In B. Biglia & C. San Martín (Eds.), *Estado de Wonderbra. Entretejiendo narrativas de feministas sobre las violencias de género* (pp. 73–83). Barcelona: Virus Press.
Mountian, I. (2009). Social imaginary for critical research. In C. Owens (Ed.), *Peer-Reviewed International Journal Annual Review of Critical Psychology* (Vol. 6, pp. 205–222). Manchester. Special Issue: Psychoanalysis.
Mountian, I. (2010). Migration and mental health: Some questions on the intersection between gender, class and race. In A. Trimboli (Ed.), *Trauma, Historia y Subjetividad* (pp. 487–489). Serie Conexiones. Buenos Aires: Editora AASM.
Mountian, I. (2012). *Políticas, Identidades e Direitos: Investigando os Enunciados da Diversidade Sexual nos Discursos Políticos nas Instâncias do Poder Legislativo em.* Minas Gerais, Research Report, PRODOC/CAPES, Belo Horizonte: UFMG.
Mountian, I. (2013a). *Cultural Ecstasies: Drugs, Gender and Social Imaginary*. London and New York: Routledge.
Mountian, I. (2013b). *Travestis e Envelhecimento*. Research Report CNPQ, edital Gênero, NUH/UFMG (Núcleo de cidadania e Direitos Humanos/Universidade Federal de Minas Gerais).
Mountian, I. (2014a). *A Critical Analysis of Public Policies on Education and LGBT Rights in Brazil*. Institute of Development Studies, Sussex University. https://opendocs.ids.ac.uk/opendocs/bitstream/handle/123456789/3614/ER61.pdf?sequence=1
Mountian, I. (2014b). Fetishism. In *Encyclopedia of Critical Psychology*. New York: Springer. http://dx.doi.org/10.1007/978-1-4614-5583-7_625
Mountian, I. (2014c). Análise de discurso e pesquisa feminista: algumas considerações sobre metodologia e ética em pesquisa. In A. F. Em Lima & N. Lara Junior (Eds.), *Metodologias de pesquisa em psicologia social crítica* (pp. 165–192). Porto Alegre: Editora Sulina.
Mountian, I. (2015a). Aspectos sobre travestilidade e envelhecimento: história, corpo e imigração. *Quaderns de Psicologia*, *17*(3), 31–44.
Mountian, I. (2015b). Psicanálise e política: reflexões nos campos de gênero e sexualidade. In J. C. Bocchi & E. O. Castro (Eds.), *Psicanálise e sociedade hoje* (Vol. 3, pp. 67–82). Curitiba and São Paulo: Editora CRV e Cultura Acadêmica Editora.
Mountian, I. (2017a). Some resources for critical research: Reflections on intersectionality, reflexivity and situationality. *Revista Psicologia Política*, *17*(40), 454–469. https://pepsic.bvsalud.org/pdf/rpp/v17n40/en_v17n40a05.pdf
Mountian, I. (2017b). Borders and margins: Debates on intersectionality for critical research. *Qualitative Research Journal*, *17*(3), 155–163.

Mountian, I. (2017c). Políticas de Drogas e intersecções de Gênero, Raça e Sexualidade. In R. Figueiredo, M. Feffermann, & R. F. Adorno (Orgs.), *Drogas & sociedade contemporânea: perspectivas para além do proibicionismo* (pp. 129–154). São Paulo: Instituto de Saúde, 2017. Coleção Temas em Saúde Coletiva, nº 22. Capítulo 3.

Mountian, I. (2019). Relações fetichizadas: a produção do Outro nas relações coloniais. *Teoría y crítica de la psicología, 13*(1), 205–220.

Mountian, I., & Gonzalez, E. C. (2019). Reflections on the theory and practice of intersectionality: Immigration and health provision services in Brazil. In S. Nayak & R. Robbins (Eds.), *Intersectionality in Social Work: Activism and Practice in Context* (pp. 92–104). London: Routledge.

Mountian, I., Monteiro, I., Vasconcelos, R., Costa, N., Sander, V., & Carneiro, J. (2012). *Travestilidade e transsexualidade e o acesso à saúde.* Report para o Ministério da Saúde. Documento não publicado.

Mountian, I., & Rosa, M. D. (2015). O outro: análise crítica de discursos sobre imigração e gênero. *Revista Psicologia USP, 26*(2), 152–160.

Mulvey, L. (1998). *Visual and Other Pleasures.* Basingstoke: Macmillan.

Munanga, K. (1990). Negritude Afro-Brasileira: perspectivas e dificuldades. *Revista de Antropologia, 33.*

Murji, K. (1999). White lines: Culture, 'race' and drugs. In N. South (Ed.), *Drugs – Cultures, Controls and Everyday Life* (pp. 49–65). London: Sage.

Musto, D. F. (1999). *The American Disease – Origins of Narcotic Control.* Oxford: Oxford University Press.

Nardi, H. C., Silveira, R. D. S., & Machado, P. S. (Org.). (2013). *Diversidade sexual, relações de gênero e políticas públicas.* Porto Alegre: Editora Sulina.

Nascimento, E. L. (2003). *O sortilégio da cor: identidade, raça e gênero no Brasil.* São Paulo: Selo Negro.

Nayak, S. (2015). *Race, Gender and Activism of Black Feminist Theory: Working with Audre Lorde.* London: Routledge.

Nayak, S. (2020, July). For women of colour in social work: Black feminist self-care practice based on Audre Lorde's radical pioneering principles. *Critical and Radical Social Work,* 1–17.

Nayak, S., & Robbins, R. (Eds.). (2019). *Intersectionality in Social Work: Activism and Practice in Context.* London: Routledge.

NHS. (2024). *Medicines Used in Mental Health England – England 2015/16 to 2023/24.* National Health System Report. https://nhsbsa-opendata.s3.eu-west-2.amazonaws.com/mumh/mumh_annual_2324_v001.html

Nieves, O. V. (1994). Lo Entre-Dicho del Discurso Lacaniano con Respecto a la Subjectividad de las Mujeres. In H. Figueroa-Sarriera, M. M. López, & M. Roman (Eds.), *Mas Alla de la Bella (In) Diferencia – Revision Post-Feminista y Otras Escrituras Posibles* (pp. 70–91). San Juan: Publicaciones Puertoriqueñas.

Nogueira, C. (2001). Construcionismo social, discurso e gênero. *Psicologia, XV*(1), 43–65.

Nogueira, F. J., & León, A. G. (2012). 'Trabalhadas no feminino': um estudo sobre corpo, desejo e prostituição travesti em Fortaleza-CE. *Revista Latinoamericana de Estudios sobre Cuerpos, Emociones y Sociedad - Relaces, 8*(4), 55–67.

Oakley, A. (1981). Interviewing women: A contradiction in terms. In H. Roberts (Ed.), *Doing Feminist Research.* London: Routledge.

Olié, J. P., Elomari, F., Spadone, C., & Lépine, J. P. (2002, September–October). Antidepressants consumption in the global population in France. *L'encephale, 28*(5 Pt 1), 411–417.

Olievenstein, C. (1989). A Dependência: Um Fenômeno Psíquico Ativo. In *A Clínica do Toxicômano – A Falta da Falta* (pp. 13–22). Porto Alegre: Artes Médicas.

Ormeño, G. R. (2012). Violência contra mulher e a mulher encarcerada sistema judiciário. *Revista da Defensoria Pública, 5*(1), 23–32.

Osborne, T. (1994). On anti-medicine and clinical reason. In C. Jones & R. Porter (Eds.), *Reassessing Foucault – Power, Medicine and the Body*. London: Routledge.
Osório, R. G., & Ferreira de Souza, P. H. G. (2012). *O Bolsa Família Depois do Brasil Carinhoso: Uma Análise do Potencial de Redução da Pobreza Extrema*. Report. Instituto de Pesquisa Econômica Aplicada (IPEA).
Oyewumi, O. (1997). *The Invention of Women: Making an African Sense of Western Gender Discourses*. Minneapolis, MN: University of Minnesota Press.
Painter, D. (2015). Postcolonial theory: Towards a worlding of critical psychology. In I. Parker (Ed.), *Handbook of Critical Psychology* (pp. 366–375). London: Routledge.
Papadopoulos, D., & Sharma, S. (2008). *Race/Matter – Materialism and Politics of Racialisation*. Retrieved March 2008, from https://orca.cardiff.ac.uk/id/eprint/27954/1/Papadopoulos%202008.pdf
Parascandola, J. (1996). The drug habit: The association of the word 'drug' with abuse in American history. In R. Potter & M. Teich (Eds.), *Drugs and Narcotics in History* (pp. 156–167). Cambridge: Cambridge University Press.
Parker, I. (1992). *Discourse Dynamics – Critical Analysis for Social and Individual Psychology*. London: Routledge.
Parker, I. (1997). Discursive psychology. In D. Fox & I. Prilleltensky (Eds.), *Critical Psychology – An Introduction*. London: Sage Publications.
Parker, I. (2002). *Discursive Resources in Discourse Unit*. In Discourse Analysis Online.
Parker, I. (2003). Lacanian social theory and clinical practice. *Psychoanalysis and Contemporary Thought*.
Parker, I. (2005). *Qualitative Psychology: Introducing Radical Research*. Maidenhead: Open University Press.
Parker, I. (2011). *Lacanian Psychoanalysis: Revolutions in Subjectivity*. London: Routledge.
Parker, I., & Pavón-Cuellar, D. (Eds.). (2014). *Lacan, Discourse, Event: New Psychoanalytic Approaches to Textual Indeterminacy*. London: Routledge.
Parker, R. (2003). Aids in Brazil. In D. Herbert & R. Parker (Eds.), *Sexuality, Politics and AIDS in Brazil: In Another World?* London: Falmer Press.
Patel, B., & Kerrigan, S. (2004). *Hungry and Homeless: The Impact of the Withdrawal of State Support on Asylum Seekers, Refugee Communities and the Voluntary Sector*. London: Refugee Council and Oxfam.
Patel, K., Buffin, J., Khurana, J., & Underwood, S. (2004). *Young Refugees and Asylum Seekers in Greater London: Vulnerability to Problematic Drug Use*. London: Great London Authority.
Pelúcio, L. (2011). "Amores perros" – Sexo, paixão e dinheiro na relação entre espanhóis e travestis brasileiras no mercado transnacional do sexo. In Adriana Piscitelli, Gláucia Oliveira Assis, & José Miguel Neto Olivar (Orgs.), *Gênero, sexo, amor e dinheiro: mobilidades transnacionais envolvendo o Brasil* (pp. 185–224). Campinas: UNICAMP/PAGU.
Pereira, V. M. (2021). *Corpos entre dobras e fronteiras: cartografia de encontros com migrantes LGBT+ em cidades mexicanas e brasileiras*. Doctorate Thesis. Programa de Pós-Graduação em Psicologia Social da Universidade do Estado do Rio de Janeiro.
Pesquisa Nacional por Amostra de Domicílios (PNAD)/Instituto Brasileiro de Geografia e Estatística (IBGE) (2011). *Síntese de Indicadores Sociais: Uma Análise das Condições de Vida da População Brasileira*. Rio de Janeiro: IBGE.
Pfeil, C. L., & Alves, R. N. (Eds.). (2024). Observatório Anderson Herzer. In *Relatório das mortes e violência contra transmasculinidades em 2023*. Curitiba: Instituto Brasileiro de Transmasculinidade.
Phillips, A. (2010). *Gender & Culture*. Cambridge: Polity Press.

Phoenix, A. (1987). Theories of gender and black families. In G. Weinger & M. Arnot (Eds.), *Gender Under Scrutiny: New Inquiries in Education* (pp. 50–63). London: Open University Press.

Phoenix, A. (2011). Transforming 'non-normative' motherhood: Retrospective accounts of transnational motherhood in serial migration. In G. M. Craig & L. O'Dell (Eds.), *Mothering on the Margins: Special Issue Editorial* (Vol. 9, No. 2, pp. 1–21). Radical Psychology.

Phoenix, A., & Seu, B. (2013). Negotiating daughterhood and strangerhood: Retrospective accounts of serial migration. *Feminism & Psychology*, *23*(3), 299–316.

Pietz, W. (1985). The problem of the fetish. *Journal of Anthropology and Aesthetics*, *9*, 5–17.

Pisciteli, A. (2008). Interseccionalidades, categorias de articulação e experiências de migrantes brasileiras. *Sociedade e Cultura*, *11*(2), 263–274.

Platero Méndez, R. (Lucas) (2014). La agencia de los Jóvenes Trans* para enfrentarse a la transfobia. *Revista Internacional de Pensamiento Político, I Época*, *9*, 183–193.

Pocahy, F. (2014). Performances of a contested body: Homo/eroticism and ageing. *Annual Review of Critical Psychology*, *11*, 219–232.

Pollard, T., & Howard, N. (2021). Mental healthcare for asylum-seekers and refugees residing in the United Kingdom: A scoping review of policies, barriers, and enablers. *International Journal of Mental Health System*, *15*, 60.

Prado, M. A. M., & Machado, F. V. (2008). *Preconceito contra homosexualidades: a hierarquia da invisivilidade*. São Paulo: Cortez editora.

Prado, M. A. M., Mountian, I., Machado, F. V., & Santos, L. C. (2010). Los movimientos LGTB y la lucha por la democratización de las jerarquias sexuales em Brasil. *Revista Digital Universitaria*, *11*(7), 1–15.

Preciado, P. B. (2020a). *An Apartment on Uranus*. London: Fitzcarraldo Editions.

Preciado, P. B. (2020b). Aprendiendo del vírus. *El País*. https://medium.com/textura/aprendendo-com-o-v%C3%ADrus-1f8542d3ed78. Also in *Sopa de Wuhan*: pensamento contemporáneo em tempos de pandemias (2020). Editorial ASPO (Aislamiento Social Preventivo y Obligatorio).

Procter, N. G. (2006). They first killed his heart (then) he took his own life. Part 2: Practice implications. *International Journal of Nursing Practice*, *12*, 42.

Programa das Nações Unidas para o Desenvolvimento (PNUD) (2011). *Relatório de Desenvolvimento Humano – Brasil 2011: Sustentabilidade e Equidade: Um Futuro Melhor para Todos*. Brasília: PNUD.

Pyne, J. (2014). The governance of gender non-conforming children: A dangerous enclosure. *Annual Review of Critical Psychology*, *11*, 79–96.

Quijano, A. (1992, December). Notas sobre a questão da identidade e nação no Peru. *Estudos Avançados*, *6*, 73–80.

Rago, M. (2013). *A Aventura de Contar-se: feminismos, escrita de si e invenções da subjetividade*. Campinas: Editora Unicamp.

Raine, P. (2001). *Women's Perspectives on Drugs and Alcohol – The Vicious Circle*. Aldershot: Ashgate.

Ramos, A. R. F. (1997). A escravidão do indígena, entre o mito e novas perspectivas de debates. *Revista de Estudos e Pesquisas*, 241–265.

Rekers, G. A. (1977). Atypical gender development and psychosocial adjustment. *Journal of Applied Behavior Analysis*, *10*(3), 559–571.

Reuter, P. (2011). *Options for Regulating New Psychoactive Drugs: A Review of Recent Experiences*. London: UK Drug Policy Commission.

Ribeiro, D. (2016). Feminismo Negro Para Um Novo Marco Civilizatório: Uma Perspectiva Brasileira. *SUR 24*, *13*(24), 99–104.

Roberts, K. (2000). Lost in the system? Disabled refugees and asylum seekers in Britain. *Disability & Society*, *15*(6), 943–948.

Robles, R., Real, T., & Reed, G. (2021). Depathologizing sexual orientation and transgender identities in psychiatric classifications. *Consortium Psychiatricum, 2*(2), 45–53.

Rodrigues, C. C. C. P., & Magri, G. (2021). Violência Contra Pessoas Transexuais: Tipos E Contextos. In Centro de Estudos de Cultura Contemporânea (CEDEC) (Ed.), *Transver O Mundo: Existências e (re)existências de travestis e pessoas trans no 1° mapeamento das pessoas trans no município de São Paulo* (pp. 161–188). São Paulo: Annablume editora.

Rodrigues, C. C. P., Aprile, M. R., & Tonhon, M. (2021). Perfil Sociodemográfico E Constituição Da Identidade De Gênero De Pessoas Transexuais No Município De São Paulo. In Centro de Estudos de Cultura Contemporânea (CEDEC) (Ed.), *Transver O Mundo: Existências e (re)existências de travestis e pessoas trans no 1° mapeamento das pessoas trans no município de São Paulo* (pp. 71–100). São Paulo: Annablume editora.

Rodrigues, L., Carneiro, N. S., & Nogueira, C. (2021). A history of scientific, medical and psychological approaches to transsexualities and their critical approach. *Saúde e Sociedade, 30*, e200768.

Rodrigues, T. (2003). *Narcotráfico – uma guerra na guerra*. São Paulo: Desatino.

Rohden, F. (2003). A construção da diferença sexual na medicina. *Cadernos de Saúde Pública*, 19(Suppl. 2), S201–S212.

Roof, J. (1996). A verdict on the paternal function: Law, the paternal metaphor, and paternity law. In W. Apollon & R. Feldstein (Eds.), *Lacan, Politics, Aesthetics* (pp. 101–126). New York: State University of New York Press.

Rosa, M. D. (1998). O Discurso e o Ato na Produção do Laço Social – Reflexões sobre a Delinqüência. In *Congresso Internacional de Psicanalise e suas Conexões – Trata-se Uma Criança*. Rio de Janeiro: Escola Lacaniana de Psicanálise.

Rosa, M. D. (1999). A Subjectivação nas Configurações Familiares da 'Pós-Modernidade. In *Psicanálise e Universidade* (pp. 79–104). Sao Paulo: Number 9/10, PUC/S.P.

Rosa, M. D. (2000). *Histórias que não se Contam – O Não-Dito e a Psicanálise com Crianças e Adolescentes*. Sao Paulo: Cabral Editora Universitária.

Rosa, M. D., & Mountian, I. (2012, March). Psychoanalytic listening of socially excluded young people. *Psychoanalysis, Culture and Society, 18*, 1–16.

Rose, G. (1995). Distance, surface, elsewhere: A feminist critique of the space of phallocentric self/knowledge. *Environment and Planning D: Society and Space, 13*, 761–781.

Rose, G. (2001). *Visual Methodologies*. London: Sage.

Rose, J. (1986). *Sexuality in the Field of Vision*. London: Verso.

Rose, N. (1994). Medicine, history and the present. In C. Jones & R. Porter (Eds.), *Reassessing Foucault – Power, Medicine and the Body*. London: Rotuledge.

Rose, N. (1999). *Governing the Soul: The Shaping of the Private Self*. London: Free Association Books.

Royal College of Psychiatrists. (2000). *Dilemmas and Choices*. London: Royal College of Psychiatrists.

Rubin, G. S. (1984/2006). *Thinking Sex: Notes for a Radical Theory of the Politics of Sexuality*. London: Routledge.

Ruggiero, V. (1999). Drug as a password and the law as a drug: Discussing the legalisation of illicit substances. In N. South (Ed.), *Drugs – Cultures, Controls and Everyday Life* (pp. 123–137). London: Sage.

Russo, M. (2011). *Migração, transformações sociais e reforma eclesial: Pastoral jesuítica e scalabriniana no Brasil da Primeira República* (pp. 7–25). Travessia: Revista do Migrante, N. 68.

Rutherford, J. (1990). The third space: Interview with Homi Bhabha. In J. Rutherford (Ed.), *Identity: Community, Culture, Difference*. London: Lawrence and Wishart.

Ryan, J. (2017). *Class and Psychoanalysis: Landscapes of Inequality*. London: Routledge.
Saavedra, L., & Nogueira, C. (2006). Memórias sobre o feminismo na psicologia: para a construção de memórias futuras. *Memorandum*, *11*, 113–127.
Saffioti, H. (1969/2013). *A mulher na sociedade de classes: mito e realidade*. Sao Paulo: Expressão Popular.
Said, E. W. (1978). *Orientalism*. London: Routledge & Kegan Paul Ltd.
Saldanha, M., & Nardi, H. C. (2016). Uma Psicologia Feminista Brasileira? Sobre destaque, apagamento e posição periférica. *Psicologia Política*, *16*(35), 35–52.
Sánchez, A., Simas, L., Diuana, V., & Larouze, B. (2020). COVID-19 nas prisões: um desafio impossível para a saúde pública? *Cadernos de Saúde Pública*, *36*(5), e00083520.
Santos, A. D. O., Schucman, L. V., & Martins, H. V. (2012). Breve histórico do pensamento brasileiro sobre relações étnico raciais. *Psicologia, Ciência e Profissão*, *32*, 166–175.
Santos, M. (2000). *Ser negro no Brasil hoje*. https://www1.folha.uol.com.br/fsp/mais/fs0705200007.htm
Santos, M. P. G. (Org.). (2018). *Comunidades terapêuticas: temas para reflexão*. Rio de Janeiro: IPEA.
Scheidlinger, S. (1982). Residential address: On scapegoating in group psychotherapy. *International Journal of Psychology*, *32*, 131–142.
Schucman, L. V. (2014). *Entre o Encardido, o Branco e o Branquíssimo. Branquitude, Hierarquia e Poder na Cidade de São Paulo*. São Paulo: Annablume.
Schwarcz, L. M. (1993). *O Espetáculo das Raças: cientistas, instituições e questão racial no Brasil 1870–1930*. São Paulo: Companhia das Letras.
Schwarcz, L. M. (2012, January). Do preto, do branco e do amarelo: sobre o mito nacional de um Brasil (bem) mestiçado. *Ciência e Cultura*, *64*(1), 48–55.
Scott, J. W. (1986, December). Gender: A useful category of historical analysis. *The American Historical Review*, *91*(5), 1053–1075.
Sedgwick, E. K. (1991). *Epistemology of the Closet*. Los Angeles: University of California Press.
Sedgwick, E. K. (1992). Epidemics of the will. In J. Crary & S. Kwinter (Eds.), *Incorporations* (pp. 582–595). New York: Zone.
Segal, L. (2015). *Straight Sex: Rethinking the Politics of Pleasure*. London: Verso.
Segato, R. L. (2006). *O Édipo Brasileiro: a dupla negação de gênero e raça*. Série Antropologia. Departamento de Antropologia, Universidade de Brasília.
Seshadri-Crooks, K. (2000). *Desiring Whiteness: A Lacanian Analysis of Race*. London: Routledge.
Shapiro, H. (1999). Dances with drugs: Pop music, drugs and youth culture. In N. South (Ed.), *Drugs – Cultures, Controls and Everyday Life* (pp. 17–35). London: Sage
Shiva, V. (1990). Reductionist science as epistemological violence. In A. Nandy (Ed.), *Science, Hegemony and Violence: A Requiem for Modernity*. Tokyo: United Nations University.
Silva, J. M., Ornat, M. J., Cabral, V., & Lee, D. (2019, July, December). 'Quando Uma Trans É Morta, Outras Mil Se Levantam!': Transnecropolítica E Transresistência No Brasil. *Geografia*, *44*(2).
Silva, T. T. (Org.). (2000). *Identidade e Diferença: A perspectiva dos Estudos Culturais*. Petrópolis: Editora Vozes.
Silvia Federic. (2013). *Silvia Federici: Gender and Democracy in the Neoliberal Agenda: Feminist Politics, Past and Present*. http://www.youtube.com/watch?v=enpTFJsswWM
Simai, S., & Baeninger, R. (2011). Racismo e sua negação: O caso dos imigrantes bolivianos em São Paulo. *Travessia: Revista do Migrante*, *68*, 49–62.

Simões, J. A. (2011). Corpo e sexualidade nas experiências de envelhecimento de homens gays em São Paulo. Em B. Trench & T. Etsuko da Costa Rosa (Eds.), *Nós e o Outro: envelhecimento, reflexões, práticas e pesquisa* (pp. 119–138). São Paulo: Instituto de Saúde.

Siqueira, M. S. (2004). *Sou Senhora – Um estudo antropológico sobre travestis na velhice*. Dissertação de Mestrado inédita, Universidade Federal de Santa Catarina.

Siqueira, M. S. (2009). *Arrasando horrores! Uma etnografia das memórias, formas de sociabilidade e itinerários urbanos de travestis das antigas*. Tese de Doutorado inédita, Universidade Federal de Santa Catarina.

Siverskog, A. (2014). "They just don't have a clue": Transgender aging and implications for social work. *Journal of Gerontological Social Work*, *57*(2–4), 386–406.

Soans, S. (2015). Cutting her nose to spite his face: Violence against women in India and the collusion of power. *Psychology of Women Section Review*, *17*, 52–65. British Psychological Society.

Soares, L. E. (2013). *A Terra Treme no país de Desigualdades e Paradoxos*. http://lareviewofbooks.org/essay/brazil-the-ground-shakes-in-the-country-of-inequalities-and-paradoxes#.UdXXlw3q-Qc.email

Soliva, T. B. (2018). Sobre o talento de ser fabulosa: os "shows de travesti" e a invenção da "travesti profissional". *Cadernos Pagu*, *53*, e185314.

Soliva, T. B. (2019, April). Sobre afetos e resistências: Uma análise da trajetória da Turma OK (Rio de Janeiro, Brasil). *Sexualidad, Salud Y Sociedad Revista Latinoamericana*, *31*, 57–80.

Soreanu, R. (2019). Supervision for our times: Countertransference and the rich legacy of the Budapest School. *American Journal of Psychoanalysis*, *79*, 329–351.

South, N. (1994). Voices from the past: Drugs and social history – From Virginia Berridge to Marek Kohn. *International Journal of Drug Policy*, *5*(4), 254–256.

South, N. (1999). Debating drugs and everyday life: Normalisation, prohibition and 'otherness'. In N. South (Ed.), *Drugs – Cultures, Controls and Everyday Life* (pp. 1–16). London: Sage.

Souza, A. C. T. C. (2015). *Drug Moms, Drug Warriors: performances de gênero e produção da (in)segurança na construção discursiva da "guerra às drogas" para a América Latina*. Master Dissertation. Pontifícia Universidade Católica do Rio de Janeiro, Instituto de Relações Internacionais.

Souza, J. (Ed.). (2006). *A Invisibilidade da Desigualdade Brasileira*. Belo Horizonte: Editora UFMG.

Souza, N. S. (1983). *Tornar-se Negro ou as Vicissitudes da Identidade do Negro Brasileiro em Ascenção Social*. Rio de Janeiro: Graal.

Souza, P. J., Ferreira, L. O. C., & Sá, J. B. (2012). Estudo Descritivo da Homofobia e Vulnerabilidade ao HIV/Aids das *Travestis* da Região Metropolitana do Recife. *Ciência e Saúde Coletiva*. ABRASCO.

Spivak, G. C. (1988). Can the subaltern speak? In C. Nelson & L. Grossberg (Eds.), *Marxism and the Interpretation of Culture* (pp. 271–313). Basingstoke: Macmillan.

Spybey, T. (1996). *Globalization and World Society*. Cambridge: Polity Press. In McMaster, Don (2003). Asylum seekers and the politics of citizenship. *Borderlands e-journal*, 2(1). https://webarchive.nla.gov.au/awa/20030825055359/borderlandsejournal.adelaide.edu.au/vol2no1_2003/mcmaster_citizen.html

Stacey, J. (1993). Untangling feminist theory. In D. Richardson & V. Robinson (Eds.), *Introducing Women's Studies* (pp. 49–73). London: Macmillan.

Stanley, L., & Wise, S. (Eds.). (1990). *Method, Methodology and Epistemology in Feminist Research Processes* in *Feminist Praxis*. London: Routledge.

Stimson, G. (1994). Can a war on drugs succeeded? In R. Coomber (Ed.), *Drugs and Drug Use in Society – A Critical Reader* (pp. 313–318). Kent: Greenwich Press.

Stimson, G. (2000). Blair declares war: The unhealthy state of British drug policy. *The International Journal of Drug Policy*, *11*, 259–264.

Suess, A. (2011). Análisis del panorama discursive alrededor de la despatologización trans: processos de transformación de los marcos interpretativos em diferentes campos sociales. In M. Missé & G. Coll-Planas (Eds.), *El Género Desordenado: Críticas em torno a la patologización de la transexualidad* (pp. 29–54). Barcelona and Madrid: Egales Editorial.
Szasz, T. (1994). The ethics of addiction. In R. Coomber (Ed.), *Drugs and Drug Use in Society – A Critical Reader* (pp. 373–382). Kent: Greenwich University Press.
Szasz, T. (1975). *Ceremonial Chemistry – The Ritual Persecution of Drugs, Addicts, and Pushers*. London: Routledge & Kegan Paul.
Tait, K., et al. (2004). *Media Image, Community Impact – Assessing the Impact of Media and Political Images of Refugees and Asylum Seekers on Community Relations in London*. London: ICAR (The Information Centre About Asylum and Refugees in the UK).
Targino, J. (2021). Interfaces entre religião, uso problemático de drogas, Moralidades e gênero em comunidades terapêuticas. In M. Fiore & T. Rui (Eds.), *Comunidades Terapêuticas No Brasil* (pp. 107–121). Working Paper Series. Social Science Research Council.
Taylor, F., & Rey, J. (1953). The scapegoat motif in society and its manifestations in a therapeutic group. *International Journal of Psychoanalysis*, *3*, 253–264.
Teixeira, F. B. (2011). Juízo e Sorte: enredando maridos e clientes nas narrativas sobre o projeto migratório das travestis brasileiras para a Itália. In Adriana Piscitelli, Gláucia Oliveira Assis, & José Miguel Neto Olivar (Orgs.), *Gênero, sexo, amor e dinheiro: mobilidades transnacionais envolvendo o Brasil* (pp. 225–262). Campinas: UNICAMP/PAGU.
Teles, M. A. A. (2007). As imigrantes bolivianas em São Paulo: o silêncio insuportável! In M. L. P. Leal, M. F. P. Leal, & R. M. C. Libório (Eds.), *Tráfico de Pessoas e Violência Sexual* (pp. 35–43). Brasília: Grupo de Pesquisa sobre Violência, Exploração Sexual e Tráfico de Mulheres, Crianças e Adolescentes – VIOLES/SER/Universidade de Brasília.
Teo, T. (2008). From speculation to epistemological violence in psychology: A critical-hermeneutic reconstruction. *Theory & Psychology*, *18*(1), 47–67. Sage Publications.
Thompson, L. (2021). Toward a feminist psychological theory of "institutional trauma". *Feminism & Psychology*, *31*(1), 99–118.
Tonelli, M. J., Maheirie, K., Perucchi, J., Mayorga, C., Mountian, I., & Prado, M. A. M. (2013). Critical social psychology in Brazil: Politics, gender, and subjects of dissidence. *Manchester: Annual Review of Critical Psychology*, *10*, 163–183.
Tosh, J. (2015). *Perverse Psychology: The Pathologization of Sexual Violence and Transgenderism*. London: Routledge.
Tosh, J. (2016). *Psychology and Gender Dysphoria – Feminist and Transgender Perspectives*. London: Routledge.
Transgender Europe (2014). *Report Monitoramento*. http://www.transrespect-transphobia.org/uploads/downloads/2014/TDOR2014/TvT-TDOR2014PR-en.pdf
Transgender Europe Monitoring Project (TGEU) (2016). *Monitoring Trans Murder Report*. http://transrespect.org/en/research/trans-murder-monitoring/
United Nations Office on Drugs and Crime. (2016). *Terminology and Information on Drugs* (3rd ed.). New York: United Nations. https://www.unodc.org/documents/scientific/Terminology_English.pdf
UN Report (2024). https://www.unodc.org/unodc/en/data-and-analysis/wdr2024-drug-market-trends.html
Ussher, J. (1991). *Women's madness: Misogyny or mental illness?* London: Harvester Wheatsheaf.
Ussher, J. M. (1998). A feminist perspective. In R. Velleman, A. Copello, & J. Maslin (Eds.), *Living with Drink – Women Who Live With Problem Drinkers* (pp. 150–161). London: Longman.

Ussher, J. M. (2018). A critical feminist analysis of madness: Pathologizing femininity through psychiatric discourse. In B. M. Z. Cohen (Ed.), *Routledge International Handbook of Critical Mental Health* (pp. 72–78). London: Routledge.
Van Haute, P., & Geysken, T. (2016). *Psicanálise sem Édipo? Uma antropologia clínica da histeria em Freud e Lacan*. São Paulo: Autêntica.
Varella, A. C. (2013). *A Embriaguez na Conquista da América: Medicina, Idolatria e Vício no México e Peru, séculos XVI e XVII*. Sao Paulo: Alameda Casa Editorial.
Vargas, E. V. (2008). Fármacos eoutros objetos sócio-técnicos: notas para uma genealogia das drogas. In B. C. Labate, S. Goulart, M. Fiore, E. MacRae, & H. Carneiro (org.), *Drogas e cultura: novas perspectivas* (pp. 41–65). Salvador: EDUFBA.
Vartabedian, J. (2014a). El alcance político de las travestilidades: acerca del potencial transgresor de las travestis. *Annual Review of Critical Psychology*, *11*, 299–317.
Vartabedian, J. (2014b). Migraciones trans: travestis brasileñas migrantes trabajadoras del sexo en Europa. *Cadernos Pagu*, *42*, 275–312.
Vergès, F. (2020). *Um Feminismo Decolonial*. São Paulo: Ubu Editora.
Vicente, M. V. (2021, November). Transgender: A useful category? Or, how the historical study of "transsexual" and "transvestite" can help us rethink "transgender" as a category. *Transgender Studies Quarterly*, *8*(4), 426–442.
Waiselfisz, J. J. (2011). *Mapa da Violência: Os Jovens do Brasil*. Brasília: Ministério da Justiça, Instituto Sangari.
Waiselfisz, J. J. (2015). *Mapa da Violência: Homicídio de mulheres no Brasil*. Brasília: Flacso.
Waiselfisz, J. J. (2016). *Mapa da Violência: Homicídios por armas de fogo no Brasil*. Brasília: Flacso.
Walusinski, O. (2014). The girls of La Salpêtrière. *Frontiers of Neurology and Neurosciences*, *35*, 65–77.
Warner, M. (1999). *The Trouble With Normal – Sex, Politics, and the Ethics of Queer Life*. Cambridge: Harvard University Press.
Warner, S. (1996). Women and high security mental hospitals. In E. Burman, G. Aitken, P. Alldred, R. Alwood, T. Billington, B. Goldberg, C. Heenan, A. Juan, G. Lopez, D. Mark, & S. Warner (Org.), *Psychology Discourse Practice: From Regulation to Resistance* (pp. 96–113). London: Taylor & Francis.
Webster, A., & Robertson, M. (2007). Can community psychology meet the needs of refugees? *The Psychologist*, *20*(3), 156–158.
White, W. L. (2004). Lessons of language: Historical perspectives on the rhetoric of addiction. In S. W. Tracy & C. J. Acker (Eds.), *Altering American Consciousness – The History of Alcohol and Drug Abuse in the United States, 1800–2000* (pp. 33–60). Minneapolis, MN: University of Massachusetts Press.
Witten, T. (2015). Elder transgender lesbians: Exploring the intersection of age, lesbian sexual identity, and transgender identity. *Journal of Lesbian Studies*, *19*(1), 73–89.
Wolf, D. L. (2002). There is no place like "home": Emotional transnationalism and the struggles of second-generation Filipinos. In P. Levitt & M. C. Waters (Eds.), *The Changing Face of Home: The Transnational Lives of the Second Generation* (pp. 255–294.). New York: Russell Sage.
World Health Organization. (1965). *lCD Classification of Mental and Behavioural Disorders Clinical Descriptions and Diagnostic Guidelines*. Geneva: World Health Organization.
World Health Organization. (1990). *lCD Classification of Mental and Behavioural Disorders Clinical Descriptions and Diagnostic Guidelines*. Geneva: World Health Organization.
World Health Organization. (1994). *Lexicon of Alcohol and Drug Terms*. Geneva: United Nations. https://www.who.int/southeastasia/health-topics/mental-health/key-terms-and-definitions-in-mental-health#addiction

World Health Organization. (1995). *ICD Classification of Mental and Behavioural Disorders Clinical Descriptions and Diagnostic Guidelines*. Geneva: World Health Organization.

Wren, K. (2007). Supporting asylum seekers and refugees in Glasgow: The role of multi-agency networks. *Journal of Refugee Studies*, *20*(3). Oxford: Oxford University Press.

Xiberras, M. (1989). *A Sociedade Intoxicada*. Lisbon: Instituto Piaget.

Young, J. (1971). *The Drugtakers – The Social Meaning of Drug Users*. London: Granada Publishing.

Yuval-Davis, N. (1997). *Gender & Nation*. London: Sage.

Zanatto, R. M. (2016). Maconha, Erva Maldita: Um Filme De Raul Roulien. In E. Macrae & W. C. Alves (Eds.), *Fumo De Angola: Canabis, racismo, resistência cultural e espiritualidade* (pp. 167–204). Salvador: EDUFBA.

Zetter, R., & Pearl, M. (2000). The minority within the minority: Refugee community-based organisations in the UK and the impact of restrictionism on asylum-seekers. *Journal of Ethnic and Migration Studies*, *26*(4), 675–697.

Zhong, W., Kremers, H. M., Yawn, B. P., Bobo, W. V., St. Sauver, J. L., Ebbert, J. O., Finney Rutten, L. J., Jacobson, D. J., Brue, S. M., & Rocca, W. A. (2014). Time trends of antidepressant drug prescriptions in men versus women in a geographically defined US population. *Archives of Women's Mental Health*, *17*, 485–492.

Zieger, S. M. (2008). *Inventing the Addict: Drugs, Race and Sexuality in Nineteenth Century in British and American Literature*. Minneapolis, MN: University of Massachusetts Press.

Zinberg, N. (1984). *Drug, Set, and Setting – The Basis for Controlled Intoxicant Use*. Yale: Yale University Press.

Zizek, S. (1992). *Enjoy Your Symptom! – Jacques Lacan in Hollywood and Out*. London: Routledge.

Zizek, S. (1998). Love thy neighbour? No, thanks! In C. Lane (Ed.), *The Psychoanalysis of Race* (pp. 154–175). New York: Columbia University Press.

Zizek, S. (1999). *The Plague of Fantasies*. London: Verso.

Zizek, S. (2001). *The One Measure of True Love Is: You Can Insult the Other*. Interview by S. Reul & T. Deichmann. London: Spiked Online.

Index

For Product Safety Concerns and Information please contact our EU representative GPSR@taylorandfrancis.com
Taylor & Francis Verlag GmbH, Kaufingerstraße 24, 80331 München, Germany

www.ingramcontent.com/pod-product-compliance
Ingram Content Group UK Ltd.
Pitfield, Milton Keynes, MK11 3LW, UK
UKHW020004200926
475702UK00015B/2461
* 9 7 8 1 0 3 2 8 7 1 6 0 8 *